U N I T   1

CONSUMER HEALTH AND SAFETY ACTIVITIES

UNIT 1

CONSUMER HEALTH AND SAFETY ACTIVITIES

PATRICIA RIZZO TONER

Just for the HEALTH of It!
Health Curriculum Activities Library

**THE CENTER FOR APPLIED
RESEARCH IN EDUCATION**

Library of Congress Cataloging-in-Publication Data

Toner, Patricia Rizzo, 1952– .
    Consumer health and safety activities / Patricia Rizzo Toner.
        p.   cm.—(Just for the health of it! ; unit 1)
    "Includes 90 ready-to-use activities and worksheets for grades
7–12."
    ISBN 0-87628-263-X
    1. Health education (Secondary)—United States—Problems,
exercises, etc.   2. Safety education—United States—Problems,
exercises, etc.   3. Consumer education—United States—Problems,
exercises, etc.   I. Title.   II. Series.
RA440.3.U5T66   1993   93-8219
613.2—dc20   CIP

The source for many of the clip art images in this book is
Presentation Task Force which is a registered trademark of New
Vision Technologies, Inc., copyright 1991.

Printed in the United States of America

10   9   8   7   6   5

ISBN 0-87628-263-X

**THE CENTER FOR APPLIED RESEARCH
IN EDUCATION**
West Nyack, NY 10994

On the World Wide Web at http://www.phdirect.com

DEDICATION

To my brothers and sisters:

Jean Ianiero of Middlesex, New Jersey
Chuck Rizzo of Gibbsboro, New Jersey
Theresa Gallagher of Stratford, New Jersey
Stephen Rizzo of Clementon, New Jersey

This dedication is in appreciation for the many
opportunities you have provided me with to jeopardize your
safety as we were growing up.
(It's one of the benefits of being the oldest.)

May you and your families enjoy good health
for many years to come. I love you.

ACKNOWLEDGMENTS

Thanks to Colleen Leh and Barb Snyder of Holland Junior High, Holland, Pennsylvania, for reviewing each activity and providing valuable feedback.

Thanks to Connie Kallback and Win Huppuch, Career and Personal Development, Prentice Hall, Englewood Cliffs, New Jersey for your valuable help and encouragement with this series.

ABOUT THE AUTHOR

Patricia Rizzo Toner, M.Ed., has taught Health and Physical Education in the Council Rock School District, Holland, PA, for over 19 years, and she has also coached gymnastics and field hockey. She is the co-author of three books: *What Are We Doing in Gym Today?, You'll Never Guess What We Did in Gym Today!,* and *How to Survive Teaching Health.* Besides her work as a teacher, Pat is also a freelance cartoonist. A member of the American Alliance for Health, Physical Education, Recreation and Dance, Pat received the Hammond Service Award, the Marianna G. Packer Book Award and was named to *Who's Who Among Students in American Colleges and Universities,* as well as *Who's Who in American Education.*

ABOUT <u>JUST FOR THE HEALTH OF IT!</u>

Just for the Health of It! was developed to give you, the health teacher, new ways to present difficult-to-teach subjects and to spark your students' interest in day-to-day health classes. It includes over 540 ready-to-use activities organized for your teaching convenience into six separate, self-contained units focusing on six major areas of health education.

Each unit provides ninety classroom-tested activities printed in a full-page format and ready to be photocopied as many times as needed for student use. Many of the activities are illustrated with cartoon figures to enliven the material and help inject a touch of humor into the health curriculum.

The following briefly describes each of the six units in the series:

Unit 1: *Consumer Health and Safety Activities* helps students recognize advertising techniques, compare various products and claims, understand consumer rights, distinguish between safe and dangerous items, become familiar with safety rules, and more.

Unit 2: *Diet and Nutrition Activities* focuses on basic concepts and skills such as the four food groups, caloric balance or imbalance, the safety of diets, food additives, and vitamin deficiency diseases.

Unit 3: *Relationships and Communication Activities* explores topics such as family relationships, sibling rivalry, how to make friends, split-level communications, assertiveness and aggressiveness, dating, divorce, and popularity.

Unit 4: *Sex Education Activities* teaches about the male and female reproductive systems, various methods of contraception ranging from abstinence to mechanical and chemical methods, sexually transmitted diseases, the immune system, pregnancy, fetal development, childbirth, and more.

Unit 5: *Stress-Management and Self-Esteem Activities* examines the causes and signs of stress and teaches ways of coping with it. Along with these, the unit focuses on various elements of building self-esteem such as appearance, values, self-concept, success and confidence, personality, and character traits.

Unit 6: *Substance Abuse Prevention Activities* deals with the use and abuse of tobacco, alcohol, and other drugs and examines habits ranging from occasional use to addiction. It also promotes alternatives to drug use by examining peer pressure situations, decision-making, and where to seek help.

To help you mix and match activities from the series with ease, all of the activities in each unit are designated with two letters to represent each resource as follows: Sex Education (SE), Substance Abuse Prevention (SA), Relationships and Communication (RC), Stress-Management and Self-Esteem (SM), Diet and Nutrition (DN), and Consumer Health and Safety (CH).

About Unit 1

Consumer Health and Safety Activities, Unit 1 in *Just for the Health of It!,* provides you with a multitude of ready-to-use activities and ideas for your Consumer Health, Safety, and First Aid units.

This resource is designed for teachers who are looking to enhance their collection of activities and ideas. It contains two main teaching tools:

- reproducibles designed for quick copying to hand out to students; and
- activities that give you ideas, games, and instructions to supplement your classroom presentation.

Use these aids to introduce a consumer health, safety, or first aid unit, to increase interest at any given point in a lesson, or to reinforce what students have learned.

An at-a-glance table of contents provides valuable help by supplying general and specific topic heads with a complete listing of activities and reproducibles. The ninety activities that make up this resource focus on the following important elements of a consumer health and safety unit:

Advertising. This section includes handouts and transparencies designed to help students understand how advertisers use a variety of methods to tout their products.

Health and Beauty Aids. This section deals with claims about skin and hair care products, mouthwashes, and diet fads. It encourages consumers to read labels carefully before buying.

Pain Relievers. Find out what the ingredients in pain relievers can and cannot do.

Quackery. This section focuses on recognizing quackery, and its effects on susceptible consumers.

Consumer Rights. Information on where you can go for help and how to get help are covered in this section.

Health Care Professionals. This section includes a game that matches health care professionals with their area of expertise.

Safety. Important elements of safety such as fire prevention, poison prevention, vehicle safety, water safety, and environmental hazards are covered with numerous handouts, games, and activities.

Accidents. Leading causes of accidental deaths at home, in school, on the job, in the neighborhood, and while involved in recreational activities as well as safety rules are emphasized in this section. Games such as Wheel of Adversity and Slamma Jamma help bring the message of safety to the students.

First Aid. This section deals with decision making concerning life-threatening emergencies.

The reproducibles and activities are designated *CH*, representing the Consumer Health and Safety component of the *Health Curriculum Activities Library*. These games, activities, puzzles, charts, and worksheets can be put directly into your lesson plans. They can be used on an individual basis or as a whole class activity.

I hope you will enjoy using these activities as much as I have.

Patricia Rizzo Toner

CONTENTS

About *Just for the Health of It!*   ix

About Unit 1   **xi**

ADVERTISING   1

Analyzing Commercials
CH-1 That's *Not* All, Folks!   2
CH-2 Name the Product   3
Activity 1: STATION BREAK   4

Advertising Techniques
Activity 2: MAKING THINGS CLEAR (Transparencies)   5
CH-3 Nostalgia   6
CH-4 Bandwagon   7
CH-5 Transfer/Fantasy   8
CH-6 Humor   9
CH-7 Sense Appeal   10
CH-8 Statistics   11
CH-9 Testimonial   12
CH-10 Ad Techniques   13
CH-11 "And Now a Word From..."   14

Price Comparison
CH-12 How Much Does It Cost?   15

HEALTH AND BEAUTY AIDS   **17**

Skin Care
CH-13 The Skin You're In   18

Mouthwashes
CH-14 Watch Your Mouth   19

Hair Care

    CH-15 Do You Care About Your Hair?   20

    CH-16 Hair Today. . .Gone Tomorrow!   21

Dieting

    Activity 3: THE DIET RIOT   22

Pain Relievers

    CH-17 What a Relief!   23

    CH-18 What a Pain!   24

QUACKERY   25

Signs of Quackery

    CH-19 Signs of Quackery   26

    CH-20 I've Got a Secret   27

Quack Devices

    CH-21 Quack Devices   28

    CH-22 Let's Make a Deal   29

Common Areas of Quackery

    CH-23 Medical Quackery   30

CONSUMER RIGHTS   31

Help for the Consumer

    CH-24 The Consumer Bill of Rights   32

    CH-25 Nader's Raiders   33

    CH-26 Nader's Raiders (cont.)   34

    CH-27 Now What Do I Do?   35

Health Care Professionals

    Activity 4: IS THERE A DOCTOR IN THE HOUSE?   36

    CH-28 Is There a Doctor in the House? Cards 1   37

    CH-29 Is There a Doctor in the House? Cards 2   38

    CH-30 Is There a Doctor in the House? Cards 3   39

CH-31 Is There a Doctor in the House? Cards 4   40

CH-32 Is There a Doctor in the House? Cards 5   41

GENERAL REVIEW ACTIVITIES   **43**

CH-33 Consumer Crossword   44

CH-34 Test Your Knowledge   45

SAFETY   **47**

Fire Prevention

CH-35 Fire Prevention Checklist   48

CH-36 Fire House   49

CH-37 Fire Escape   50

Poison Prevention

Activity 5: POISON PATROL   51

CH-38 Poison Patrol Answer Sheet   52

CH-39 Pick Your Poison   53

Auto Safety

CH-40 On the Lookout!   54

CH-41 Seat Belts *Do* Save Lives   55

Bicycle Safety

CH-42 Are You a Safe Rider?   56

CH-43 Bike Safety Survey   57

Water Safety

CH-44 Water Safety Unscramble   53

Environmental Safety

Activity 6: ENVIRONMENTAL HAZARDS   59

Activity 7: IT'S HAZARDOUS TO YOUR HEALTH   60

ACCIDENTS 61

Causes of Accidents

CH-45 I've Fallen and I Can't Get Up!   62
CH-46 It Was an Accident!   63
CH-47 There's No Place Like Home   64

Safety Rules

CH-48 Be Careful, You'll Poke Your Eye Out!   65
CH-49 An Ounce of Prevention   66
Activity 8: WHEEL OF ADVERSITY   67
Figure 1. Classroom Setup   68
CH-50 Wheel of Adversity Game Wheel   69
CH-51 Wheel of Adversity Desk Signs   70
CH-52 Wheel of Adversity Desk Signs   71
CH-53 Wheel of Adversity Question Cards   72
CH-54 Wheel of Adversity Question Cards   73
CH-55 Wheel of Adversity Question Cards   74
CH-56 Wheel of Adversity Accident Cards   75
CH-57 Wheel of Adversity Accident Cards   76
CH-58 What's Wrong With This Picture?   77
CH-59 What's Wrong With This Picture?   78
Activity 9: KNOW THE RULES   79
CH-60 Know the Rules Gameboard   80
CH-61 Know the Rules Game Cards   81
CH-62 Know the Rules Game Cards   82
CH-63 Know the Rules Game Cards   83
CH-64 Make Your Own Game Cards   84
CH-65 Safety Toons   85
Activity 10: SLAMMA JAMMA   86
CH-66 Slamma Jamma Cards   87
CH-67 Slamma Jamma Checklist   88

FIRST AID 89

Animals and Insects

CH-68 Bites and Stings   90
CH-69 Bee Safe   91

Emergency Procedures

Activity 11: RESCUE 911   92

CH-70 This Is an Emergency!   93

CH-71 Be a Lifesaver!   94

CH-72 Split-Second Decision   95

CH-73 Split-Second Decision Worksheet   96

General Knowledge

CH-74 Test Your First Aid I.Q.   97

CH-75 Emergency Terms You Should Know   98

CH-76 A Matter of Life and Death (Strokes)   99

CH-77 A Matter of Life and Death (Heart Attacks)   100

CH-78 A Matter of Life and Death (Choking)   101

CH-79 Emergency Handbook   102

CH-80 Emergency Handbook (2)   103

ANSWER KEYS TO REPRODUCIBLES   **105**

ADVERTISING

- **Analyzing Commercials**

- **Advertising Techniques**

- **Price Comparison**

THAT'S NOT ALL, FOLKS! (CH-1)

DIRECTIONS: Watch one (1) hour of cartoons, either after school or Saturday mornings. Write down the information requested on the chart below. A stopwatch and calculator will be helpful in completing this assignment. When you are finished, report your findings back to the class and compare them to your classmates' findings.

CARTOON	# OF MINUTES	COMMERCIAL	TYPE OF PRODUCT (Food, action figure, doll, candy, etc.)	# OF SECONDS OR MINUTES

Percentage of hour devoted to commercials _____%
Percentage of commercial time devoted to:

TOYS _____% FOOD _____% CANDY _____% OTHER _____%

NAME THE PRODUCT (CH-2)

DIRECTIONS: Listed below are some advertising slogans, or descriptions. Can you name the products described? Place your answer in the blank.

_____ 1. The soft drink that states, "You got the right one, baby…uh, huh!"

_____ 2. A bunny appears on the TV screen as the announcer says, "It keeps going and going and going…"

_____ 3. "Soup so big, it eats like a meal."

_____ 4. A family fights over waffles shouting, "Leggo my _____ !"

_____ 5. "JUST DO IT!"

_____ 6. "There's always room for _____ ?" this gelatin dessert.

_____ 7. A fast food restaurant that says you can have it "your way, right away!"

_____ 8. A man needing mustard for his sandwich rolls down the window to his Rolls Royce and asks, "Pardon me, but would you have any _____ ?"

_____ 9. A car company that asks, "Have you driven a _____ , lately?"

_____ 10. A car company where its buyers jump into the air and exclaim, "I love what you do for me, _____ "

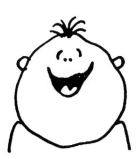

"Ummm…..
     is the answer
     Wendy's ?"

ACTIVITY 1: STATION BREAK

Concept/ Description: Advertisers use various methods to sell their products to consumers.

Objective: To demonstrate an understanding of advertising techniques by creating a commercial.

Materials: Will depend on type of ad students choose.

Directions:
1. Divide students into groups of four or five and assign them an advertising technique.
2. Have students devise their own commercial using the advertising method assigned to them.
3. Have the groups perform their commercials for the class and have the class try to guess the method used.
4. Discuss the methods that are most appealing to class members. Ask them to speculate as to why there are so many different advertising methods. (People have different tastes, and advertisers try to reach all types of target audiences.)

"And now a word from our sponsor...."

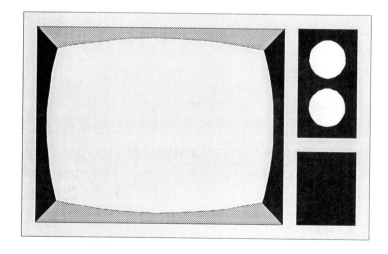

ACTIVITY 2: MAKING THINGS CLEAR

Concept/   Advertisers use various methods to sell their products to con-
Description: sumers.

Objective: To understand and give examples of some common advertising
techniques.

Materials: Overhead transparencies of advertising tcchniques (CH-3 to
CH-9)
Overhead projector
Screen or blank wall

Directions: 1. Prior to class, have sheets (CH-3 to CH-9) made into transparencies using a thermal copy machine.
2. If that is unavailable, have the sheets laminated and display
them at various points in the room.
3. Show each advertising method and ask students to give
examples of commercials that fit each category.

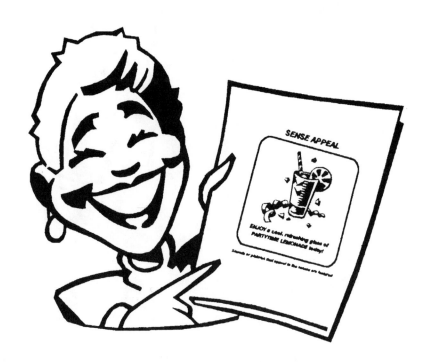

At Chadwick Hospital, we treat our patients the way they treated patients back in the good old days.

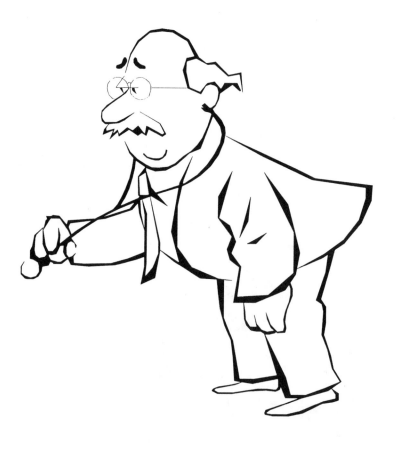

Plainfolks, back-to-nature, just the way grandma used to make it, back in the good old days.

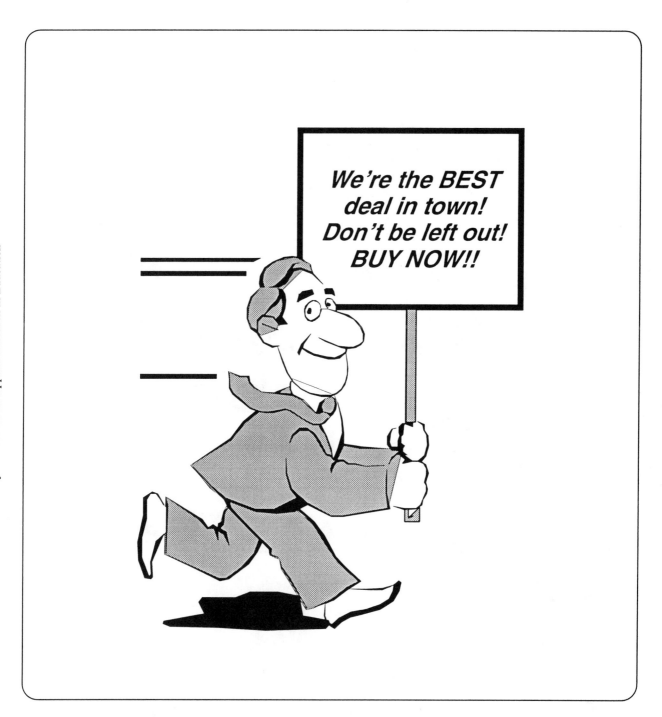

**Everyone who is anyone is buying this product.
Don't be the only one without it. Don't be left out!**

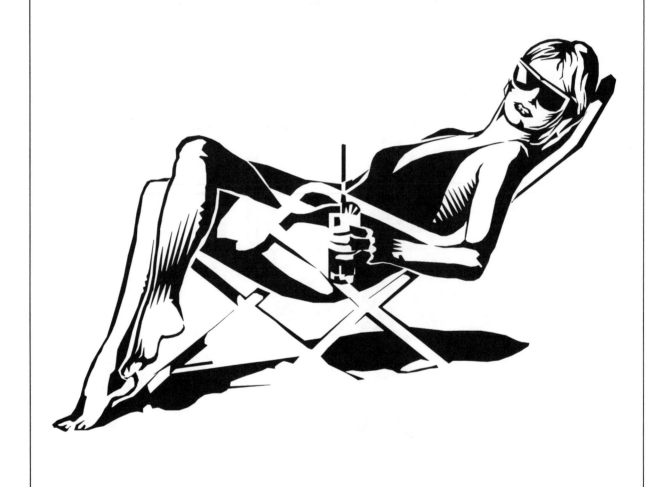

MEN:

TO MEET THE WOMAN OF YOUR DREAMS...
USE FRESHMINT TOOTHPASTE!

Superheros, white knights, green giants, super athletes, beautiful people, rich people are featured. Advertisers hope that the consumer will tend to transfer these qualities to the products and themselves and purchase the item.

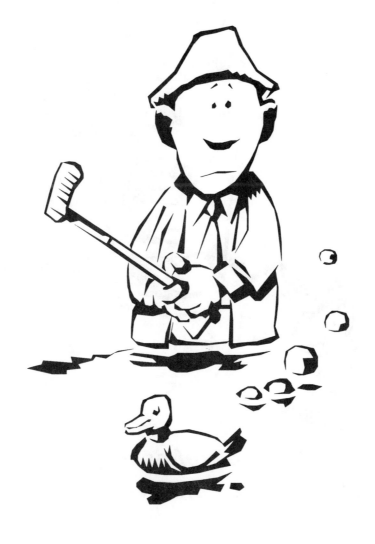

Is your golf game getting you down?
CALL ACTION GOLF CENTER!

People tend to remember an ad if it makes them laugh and may purchase the product because of the positive association with it.

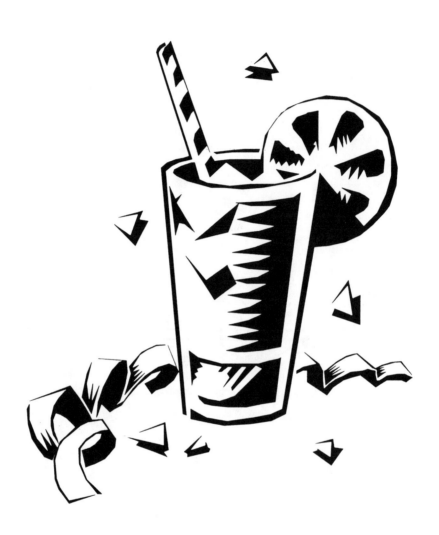

ENJOY a cool, refreshing glass of PARTYTIME LEMONADE today!

Sounds or pictures that appeal to the senses are featured.

"3 out of 4 doctors in 7 out of 10 hospitals recommend that 87% of their patients who suffer from the #1 leading ailment read the magazine that offers over 43 million ideas for 16.3% of....."

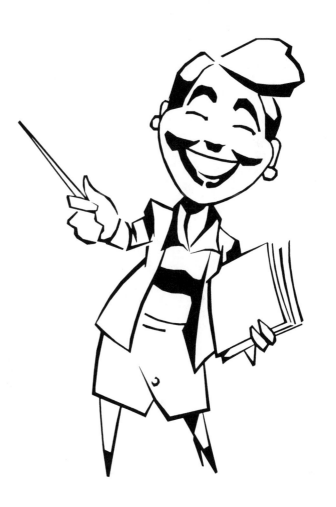

People tend to be impressed with "facts" and statistics even if they have little or no meaning.

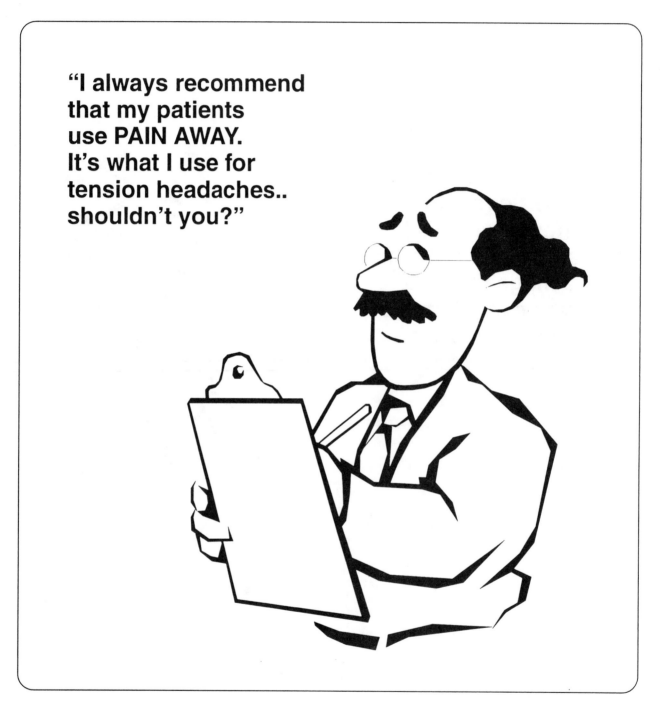

"I always recommend that my patients use PAIN AWAY. It's what I use for tension headaches.. shouldn't you?"

©1993 by The Center for Applied Research in Education

Important or well-known people testify that they use the product and so should you.

AD TECHNIQUES (CH-10)

DIRECTIONS: Listed below are some commonly used advertising methods. Match the ad described with the technique by placing the correct letter in the blank.

TECHNIQUES:

NOSTALGIA: Plainfolks, back-to nature, just the way grandma used to make it, back in the good old days.

BANDWAGON: Everyone who is anyone is buying this product. Don't be the only one without it. Don't be left out!

TRANSFER/FANTASY: Superheros, white knights, green giants, super athletes, beautiful people, rich people are featured. Advertisers hope that the consumer will tend to transfer these qualities to the products and themselves and purchase the item.

HUMOR: People may tend to remember an ad if it makes them laugh and may purchase the product because of the positive association with it.

SENSE APPEAL: Sounds or pictures that appeal to the senses are featured.

STATISTICS: People tend to be impressed with "facts" and statistics even if they have little or no meaning.

TESTIMONIAL: Important or well-known people testify that they use the product and so should you.

MATCHING:

_____1. "Lose weight the way 6 million Americans have. It's the method 3 out of 4 doctors recommend."

_____2. A cool, sparkling soft drink sits next to a hot, sizzling cheeseburger.

_____3. A famous actor says that he buys a product and recommends it to everyone.

_____4. Lemonade is served on the back porch of a house situated near an old fishin' pond.

_____5. "Buy your next car at Crazy Joe's, where everyone gets the best deal around!"

_____6. A person falls down a flight of steps and says, "It's the kind of soft drink you could fall for!"

_____7. A woman driving in her new convertible runs her hands through her beautiful blonde hair to show how great Shimmer Shampoo works.

A. Humor
B. Sense Appeal
C. Transfer/Fantasy
D. Testimonial
E. Nostalgia
F. Statistics
G. Bandwagon

"AND NOW A WORD FROM..." (CH-11)

DIRECTIONS: Using one of the advertising techniques listed below, design a magazine ad for the product shown. Refer to the AD TECHNIQUES worksheet for an explanation of each advertising type.

Check the advertising technique you will use:

_____ NOSTALGIA   _____ SENSE APPEAL
_____ BANDWAGON   _____ STATISTICS
_____ TRANSFER/FANTASY   _____ TESTIMONIAL
_____ HUMOR

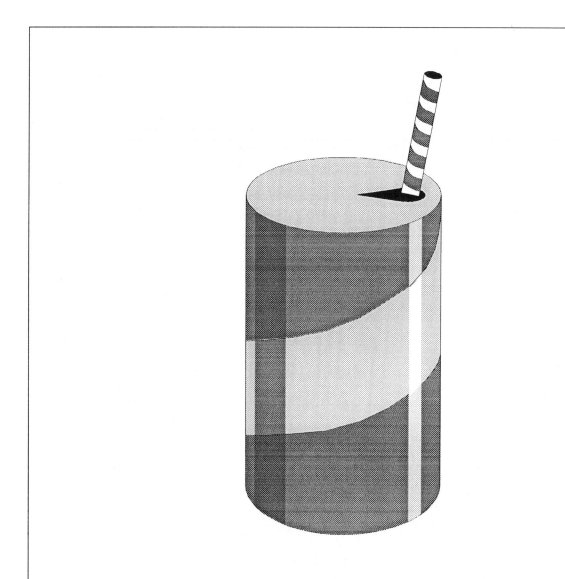

©1993 by The Center for Applied Research in Education

Name _____ **Date** _____

HOW MUCH DOES IT COST? (CH-12)

DIRECTIONS: One of the many factors that influences consumers to purchase goods or services is PRICE. Price is influenced by several things. Brand names cost more because the cost of advertising is passed on to the consumer. The size of the product affects the price, and where the product is sold (department store, grocery store, convenience store, etc.) affects the price. Choose any product and compare it in the ways listed below. Report your findings back to the class.

PRODUCT _____

PRODUCT NAME	BRAND (B) OR GENERIC (G)?	STORE NAME	TYPE OF STORE	UNIT PRICE

HEALTH AND BEAUTY AIDS

- **Skin Care**

- **Mouthwashes**

- **Hair Care**

- **Dieting**

- **Pain Relievers**

THE SKIN YOU'RE IN (CH-13)

DIRECTIONS: Take the skin quiz below to discover how much you know about your skin. Write an *X* in the correct box.

	TRUE	FALSE
1. The largest organ in the body is the skin.	☐	☐
2. The most effective over-the-counter (OTC) treatment for acne is to use products that contain benzoyl peroxide.	☐	☐
3. Medicated soaps are a great treatment for acne because the medication seeps into the pores.	☐	☐
4. Acne occurs when the skin pores become clogged with dead skin cells and dirt.	☐	☐
5. Products containing lanolin are best to use if you have acne.	☐	☐
6. Acne is caused by eating fatty foods and chocolate.	☐	☐
7. Antibacterial soaps are excellent in the treatment of acne.	☐	☐
8. If you have acne, it is best to use water-based cosmetics or no cosmetics at all.	☐	☐
9. The most active sebaceous (oil-producing) glands are located in the scalp.	☐	☐
10. Look for products containing sulfur, resorcinol, or salicylic acid to treat the more severe cases of acne.	☐	☐

WATCH YOUR MOUTH (CH-14)

DIRECTIONS: Read the labels on various brands of mouthwashes. For each container below, list a brand of mouthwash and the amount of alcohol each contains. Mouthwashes with alcohol can actually dry out the mouth and may even contribute to infection.

1. %

2. 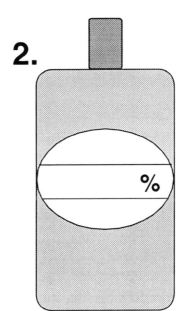 %

3. 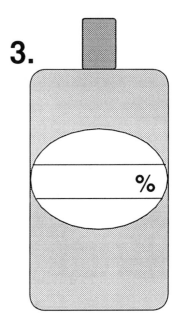 %

4. 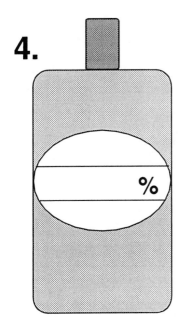 %

5. 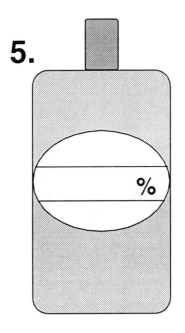 %

6. 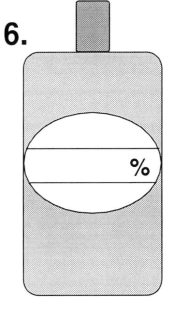 %

DO YOU CARE ABOUT YOUR HAIR? (CH-15)

DIRECTIONS: How much do you know about hair care? Place a *T* for TRUE or an *F* for FALSE in the blank.

_____ 1. Only shampoos that produce a great deal of suds or lather clean well.

_____ 2. Using mild dishwashing liquid to shampoo your hair will not damage your hair.

_____ 3. Ingredients such as egg, lemon juice, and herbs are of no special benefit to the hair.

_____ 4. Certain types of shampoo will mend split ends.

_____ 5. Surfactants are chemicals in shampoo that can grab hold of dirt and oil and then attract water to wash them away.

_____ 6. Shampoos for oily hair contain less detergent than those for dry hair.

_____ 7. Washing your hair several times per week, no matter which shampoo you use, generally keeps dandruff under control.

_____ 8. If you do experience "flaking" of the scalp, a shampoo containing selenium may help.

_____ 9. For shampoos to be safe, they should be "pH balanced."

_____ 10. To have clean, "healthy" hair, you need to purchase a well-known hair care system.

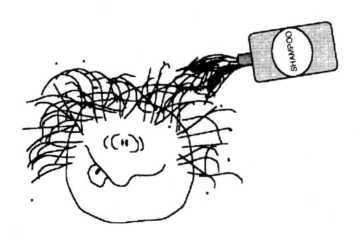

©1993 by The Center for Applied Research in Education

HAIR TODAY...GONE TOMORROW! (CH-16)

DIRECTIONS: There are hundreds of "surefire cures" for baldness, most of which promise a great deal, but deliver very little. In a group of three or four, research the methods and products listed below, and add any others that you may know of.

PRODUCT OR METHOD	BRIEF DESCRIPTION	COST	ADVANTAGES OR DISADVANTAGES
Minoxidil			
Hair Transplants			
Hair Club for Men			
Colored Scalp Sprays			
Hair Weaves			
Toupees			

ACTIVITY 3: THE DIET RIOT

Concept/ Description: Diet aids represent one of the most popular areas of quackery. The promoters play on people's need to be fit, trim, and energetic. Some products include energy restorers, vitamin supplements, diets, body builders, and pep pills.

Objective: To examine various products and diets that may be fraudulent.

Materials: In the weeks preceding this lesson, collect (or have students supply you with) pamphlets, actual products, videos, etc., promoting diets, diet aids, and vitamin supplements, such as:

KLB-6
Herbal-Life
10-Day Fast
Nutri-System
Slim Fast
Cybergenics

The Bran Diet
9-Day Wonder
Weight Watchers
Jenny Craig
Lean Line

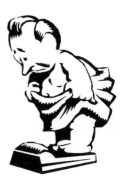

Directions:
1. Assign small groups a particular product or service such as the ones listed above.
2. Have each group research the products or services and report back to the class.
3. Reports should attempt to answer the following questions:
   a. Is the product nutritionally balanced?
   b. Does the product or service recommend exercise?
   c. Is the cost manageable by the average consumer?
   d. How long are you supposed to use the product or service?
   e. How convenient is this product?
   f. Do you think this is a valuable product or service? Why or why not? Explain in detail.
   g. Would you recommend this product or service to a friend?
4. After all groups have presented their information, compile a list of recommended and not recommended products and services.

Variation: Invite representatives from various companies that offer the product or service to speak to your classes.

WHAT A RELIEF! (CH-17)

DIRECTIONS: Look at various bottles of pain relievers and list all the different ingredients below. Write the ingredients anywhere in the space around the pictures. Circle any ingredient and write a paragraph on the effect that ingredient has on the body. In the space provided, list the name brands that have the ingredient you chose.

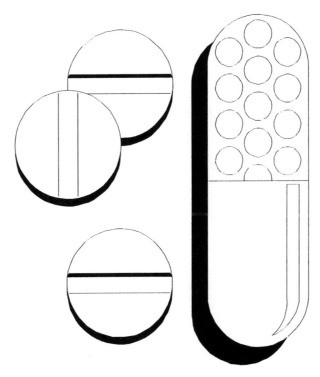

Paragraph

_____
_____
_____
_____
_____

Products Containing Ingredient:

_____ _____

_____ _____

_____ _____

_____ _____

Name _____ **Date** _____

WHAT A PAIN! (CH-18)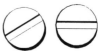

DIRECTIONS: Go to a local supermarket or drug store and check the aisle that displays pain relievers. Look at the labels and write the names of the products in the proper category: either acetaminophen, acetylsalicylic acid (aspirin), or ibuprofen. A description of each type of pain reliever is provided below.

ACETAMINOPHEN. This product lowers fever and reduces pain, but it doesn't reduce swelling. Swelling can be the result of arthritis, some headaches, and some strains and sprains.

ACETYLSALICYLIC ACID (Aspirin). This product can reduce swelling, relieve pain, and lower fever. Aspirin should NEVER be used by children with chicken pox or flu because it may contribute to Reye's syndrome, which can cause possible brain damage and death.

IBUPROFEN. This product is even stronger than aspirin in reducing swelling and inflammation. It is also irritating to the stomach.

ACETAMINOPHEN	ACETYLSALICYLIC ACID	IBUPROFEN

©1993 by The Center for Applied Research in Education

QUACKERY

- **Signs of Quackery**

- **Quack Devices**

- **Common Areas of Quackery**

SIGNS OF QUACKERY (CH-19)

How do you tell if a product is a legitimate deal or quackery? Listed below are some questions to ask yourself when purchasing a questionable item. If you can answer "YES" to any of the questions, quackery is likely to be involved.

1. Is the product offered as a "secret" remedy?

2. Is the product "not available elsewhere"?

3. Is the sponsor claiming to be fighting the medical profession that does not accept his or her "wonderful" discovery?

4. Is the product sold door-to-door by so-called "health advisors"?

5. Are the products called "miracle" drugs, devices, diets, anti-aging creams, etc.?

6. Do the promoters tell you of the wonderful miracles their products or services have done for others?

7. Are the products or services good for a wide variety of real or imagined illnesses and ailments?

8. Does the promised result seem too good to be true?

©1993 by The Center for Applied Research in Education

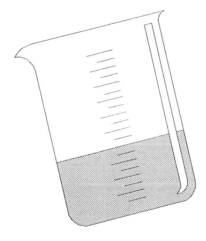

**Dr. Demento's
Miracle Bunion
Cure
ONLY
$19.95**

I'VE GOT A SECRET! (CH-20)

DIRECTIONS: Shown below is a "quack" advertisement for a fictitious product. Circle all the things in this ad that would make it quackery. Refer to the SIGNS OF QUACKERY (CH-19) list if you need help.

The AMAZING, STUPENDOUS
"MY SECRET"
Miracle Potion

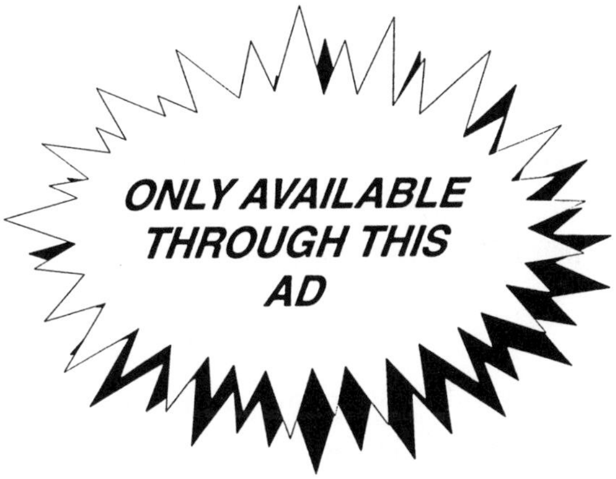

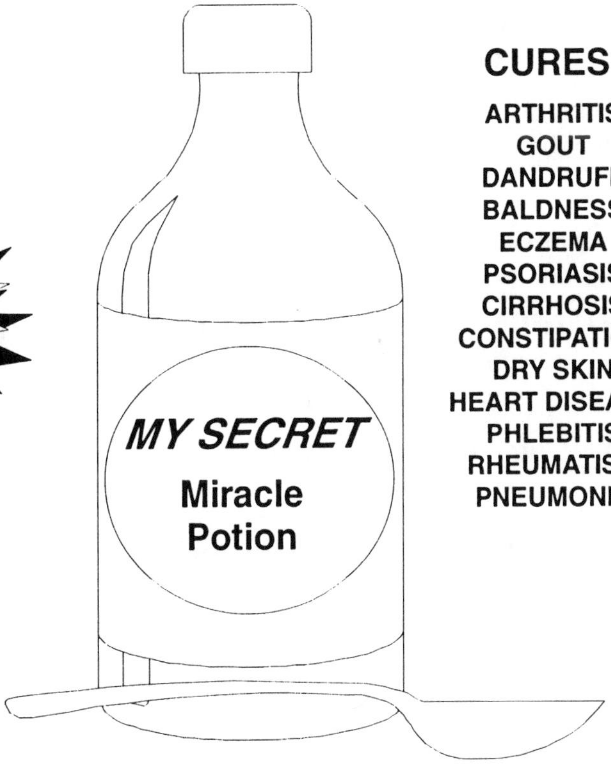

CURES:

ARTHRITIS
GOUT
DANDRUFF
BALDNESS
ECZEMA
PSORIASIS
CIRRHOSIS
CONSTIPATION
DRY SKIN
HEART DISEASE
PHLEBITIS
RHEUMATISM
PNEUMONIA

ONLY AVAILABLE THROUGH THIS AD

MY SECRET
Miracle Potion

Mr. John M. of Santa Clara says, "I love "MY SECRET," it's a miracle in a bottle..."

"My Secret" is a new product that has performed miracles for all my clients. The American Medical Association is currently fighting to keep my product off the market, but I am so convinced you'll love the results, that I am practically giving away my potion for only

$39.95 per bottle.

QUACK DEVICES (CH-21)

For thousands of years people have fallen prey to health quackery. It is big business and can provide a considerable income for the so-called "health gurus" who promote their devices. Unfortunately, use of such products can delay proper treatment and drain the pocketbook. Listed below are the categories for quack medical devices. If you think you are a victim of quackery, you can get help (see CH-25 and CH-26).

MEDICAL DEVICE QUACKERY CATEGORIES:

1. **Diagnostic and Treatment Machines:** Machines with impressive looking dials, lights, and sounds. Sometimes they are deliberately designed to look like an actual scientific device.

2. **Radiating Devices:** Devices that appear to give off radiation, or new types of "medical rays."

3. **Electricity and magnetism:** Various types of machines that produce electric shock or generate magnetic force.

4. **Light and Sound Machines:** Lights and sounds that are supposed to "cure" illness.

5. **Air Purifiers and Negative Ion Generators:** Air purifiers that are promoted for treating viral or bacterial diseases.

6. **Vibrating Devices:** Vibrators that have claimed to cure all types of ailments.

7. **Devices for Erasing the Ravages of Time:** Devices that supposedly could eliminate wrinkles and the effects of aging.

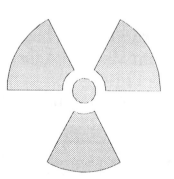

LET'S MAKE A DEAL (CH-22)

DIRECTIONS: Refer to the QUACK DEVICES handout (CH-21) and choose a category. In the space provided, design a quack device. Draw the device and explain in detail what the device will do. Be sure to include the price.

NEW

MEDICAL QUACKERY (CH-23)

DIRECTIONS: Unscramble the words to form a list of terms dealing with common forms of medical quackery.

1. ACCENR   abnormal growth of cells

2. LPCEAOB   substance that has no medical value

3. SITIRHTRA   condition that causes aching and pain in the joints

4. GGANI   growing old

5. EIWHGT   heaviness

6. DIAS   acquired immune deficiency syndrome

7. LDABSSNE   hair loss

8. LESRWKNI   caused by aging or ultraviolet rays

9. DOOF DAFS   schemes that feature food, diets, or diet supplements

10. STUB VDEELPORES   breast enhancers

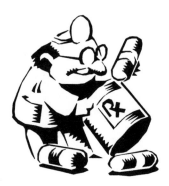

"I bet this stuff will grow hair..."

©1993 by The Center for Applied Research in Education

CONSUMER RIGHTS

- Help for the Consumer

- Health Care Professionals

THE CONSUMER BILL OF RIGHTS (CH-24)

As a consumer, you have certain basic rights. In 1962, the Consumer Bill of Rights was introduced by President Kennedy. Since the original bill, former President Nixon and former President Ford have added additional rights. The Consumer Bill of Rights is outlined below:

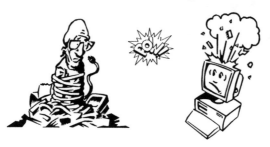

The Right to Safety

You are protected from the sale of dangerous products.

The Right to Choose

You have the right to select from goods and services at competitive prices.

The Right to Be Informed

You are protected from false advertising and you have the right to ask for all the facts you need to make decisions.

The Right to Be Heard

You have the right to speak out when you are not satisfied. You have the right to help in making consumer laws.

The Right to Redress

You have the right to have a problem corrected or solved if you have not been treated fairly.

The Right to Consumer Education

You have the right to learn the skills to make you a wise consumer.

NADER'S RAIDERS (CH-25)

If you encounter a problem with a product, the first step is to go to the source. Return it to the place of purchase and see if you can get help or advice on what to do next. If this does not help, then you may need to go for help. There are three basic types of groups that help consumers with problems: business groups, government agencies, and consumers groups. A well-known consumer group is "Nader's Raiders," the Public Interest Research Group.

Ralph Nader is a consumer advocate who has been in the public eye for many years. He speaks out for the public. He and his group, "Nader's Raiders," have done a great deal to support consumer interests. Listed below are places to go for help if you have a consumer concern. After studying the list, try the NOW WHAT DO I DO? worksheet. (See CH-27).

1. **The Better Business Bureau (BBB).** This is a non-profit organization that offers many services. The BBB gives general information to the public on products and services. It keeps records of the way in which local businesses handle complaints, and background information about the business as well. The BBB will accept written complaints and will contact a local firm on your behalf. It will also handle cases involving false advertising.

2. **TV or Radio Stations.** Sometimes local TV or radio stations offer consumer "hotline" services. These often are very helpful because of the powerful effect of adverse publicity.

3. **Small-Claims Court.** These court procedures are usually quick, inexpensive, and informal. You usually do not need a lawyer. These courts deal with claims that are between $100 and $3000.

4. **Consumer Affairs Offices.** There are state, county, and city offices in most states. They have a large selection of educational materials and information available.

5. **Private Consumer Groups.** These are groups that help individual consumers with complaints. You can contact your local consumer affairs office to get more information about groups in your area.

NADER'S RAIDERS *(continued)* (CH-26)

6. Government Agencies. The federal government has a number of specialized agencies that deal with health-related products and services. Some are listed below:

- The Consumer Product Safety Commission. The CPSC protects consumers against the making and sale of dangerous toys, games, appliances, etc. Call 1-800-638-2772 for information.

- The Consumer Information Center. The CIC distributes information to consumers. The address is: Consumer Information Center
   Pueblo, Colorado 81009

- The Food and Drug Administration. The FDA makes sure that food is safe and that it is labeled correctly. It also makes sure that cosmetics are safe and that drugs are labeled and safe.

- Federal Trade Commission. The FTC prevents the unfair, false, or deceptive advertising of consumer products and services.

- The Food and Safety Quality Service. The FSQS of the Department of Agriculture makes sure that meat and poultry are safe and labeled properly.

"There is something wrong with this cheese!!!"

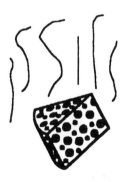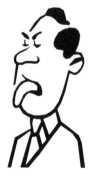

Name _____ **Date** _____

NOW WHAT DO I DO? (CH-27)

DIRECTIONS: For each scenario listed below, match it with the agency or group that is most likely able to help. Place the letter of the BEST choice in the blank. Refer to the worksheet "NADER'S RAIDERS" (CH 25-26) for help in determining what each agency does.

a. BBB (Better Business Bureau)
b. Small-Claims Court
c. CIC (Consumer Information Center)
d. CPSC (Consumer Product Safety Commission)
e. FDA (Food and Drug Administration)
f. FTC (Federal Trade Commission)
g. FSQS (Food and Safety Quality Service)

_____ 1. The head fell off of the doll you bought for your sister, exposing a sharp, jagged piece of metal.

_____ 2. A local business placed an ad in a local paper, and you believe it is false advertising.

_____ 3. You want to check out the complaint record of a local business.

_____ 4. You would like a catalogue of consumer information.

_____ 5. You have a severe skin rash and blistering after using a new brand of deodorant.

_____ 6. After taking your new car to a car wash, you notice about $500 worth of damage to the paint and trim. The owner refuses to pay for repairs, but you are certain that it is the fault of the car wash.

_____ 7. The electric razor that you bought gives you an electric shock each time you attempt to use it.

_____ 8. You purchase a can of fruit that is contaminated by worms.

_____ 9. A new type of eye mascara causes a burning sensation in your eyes.

_____ 10. You purchase chicken that does not look or taste like chicken. You believe that the package is labeled incorrectly.

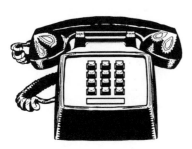

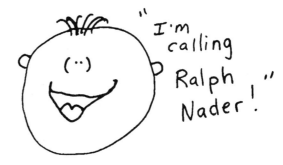

ACTIVITY 4: IS THERE A DOCTOR IN THE HOUSE?

Concept/ Description: There are many health care professionals and consumers should be aware of their area of expertise.

Objective: Be the first group to match all the jobs to their descriptions.

Materials: IS THERE A DOCTOR IN THE HOUSE? cards (CH-28 to CH-32)
Flat playing surface (floor, table, etc.)

Directions:
1. Reproduce the game cards so that each group of four students has a set.
2. If possible, laminate the cards so they will last.
3. Cut the sets of cards and shuffle them.
4. Divide the class into groups of approximately four.
5. Give each group a set of shuffled cards.
6. On the signal, have the groups match the profession to the description by placing the cards side by side.
7. The first group to complete the task correctly is declared the winner.
8. Discuss the various professions.

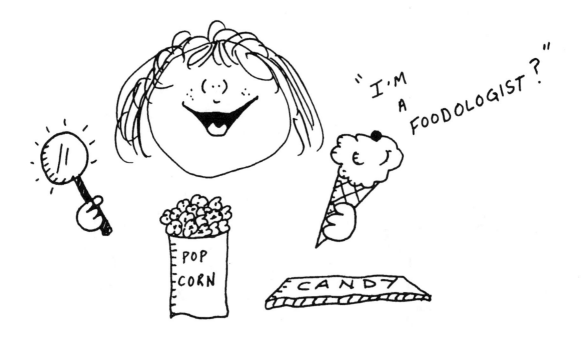

IS THERE A DOCTOR IN THE HOUSE? Cards (CH-28)

ALLERGIST	**Diagnoses and treats asthma, hay fever, and other allergies.**
ANESTHESIOLOGIST	**Administers painkilling drugs during surgery.**
CARDIOLOGIST	**Diagnoses and treats heart diseases.**
DERMATOLOGIST	**Diagnoses and treats skin diseases.**

ENDOCRINOLOGIST	**Diagnoses and treats endocrine gland problems.**
GASTRO-ENTEROLOGIST	**Treats stomach and intestinal disorders.**
GYNECOLOGIST	**Diagnoses and treats problems of the female reproductive system.**
NEUROLOGIST	**Diagnoses and treats problems of the nervous system.**

OBSTETRICIAN	**Specializes in all areas of childbirth.**
OPHTHALMOLOGIST	**Diagnoses and treats eye problems.**
ORTHOPEDIC SURGEON	**Performs surgery on bones and joints.**
OTO-LARYNGOLOGIST	**Treats disorders of the ears, nose, and throat.**

OTOLOGIST	**Diagnoses and treats ear problems.**
PATHOLOGIST	**Does lab tests of body tissues and fluids to study the causes of illness and death.**
PEDIATRICIAN	**Specializes in the medical care of children.**
PLASTIC SURGEON	**Treats skin and soft-tissue deformities and performs surgery to improve features.**

PSYCHIATRIST	**Specializes in mental and emotional disorders.**
RADIOLOGIST	**Uses X rays and radium therapy.**
THORACIC SURGEON	**Performs surgery on the chest and lungs.**
UROLOGIST	**Treats disorders of the urinary tract and the male reproductive system.**

GENERAL
REVIEW
ACTIVITIES

CONSUMER CROSSWORD (CH-33)

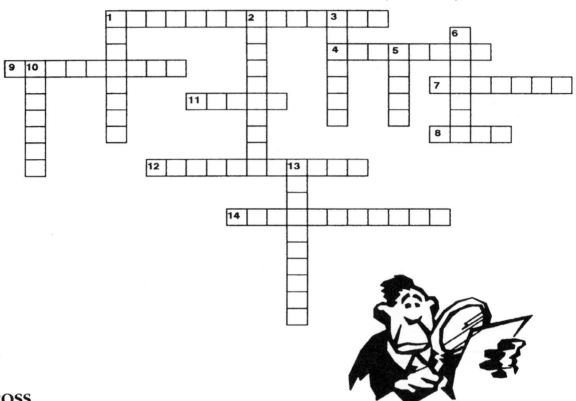

©1993 by The Center for Applied Research in Education

ACROSS

1. A product that helps control underarm perspiration
4. A person who buys or uses goods or services
7. An effective OTC ingredient to fight acne is _____ peroxide
8. A skin disorder
9. Bad breath
11. Cost or _____
12. All the methods a manufacturer uses to get your attention for its product
14. A method of advertising where a famous or important person tells how great the product is and that you, too, should use it

DOWN

1. A person who speaks out for a position
2. A compound in shampoo that attracts oil and water and cleans your hair
3. An ingredient to avoid in mouthwash since too much can dry out the mouth
5. The oil secreted from the glands of the skin and scalp
6. Not a "brand name" drug
10. Acetylsalicylic acid
13. A method of advertising that sometimes uses insignificant facts and figures to tout the product

Name _____ **Date** _____

TEST YOUR KNOWLEDGE (CH-34)

DIRECTIONS: How knowledgeable are you about consumer health? Take the test below to find out. Place a *T* for TRUE or an *F* for FALSE in the blank to the left.

_____ 1. Certain types of gum can freshen your breath and whiten your teeth.

_____ 2. It is unsafe to use a generic brand of aspirin because it might not contain the correct ingredients.

_____ 3. If statistics, such as "three out of four doctors recommend this product," are used in a commercial, then the product would definitely be good.

_____ 4. The best way for a woman to keep herself clean is to use feminine deodorant sprays and douche regularly.

_____ 5. Using mouthwashes containing alcohol can actually dry out the mouth and possibly contribute to infection.

_____ 6. The best acne medications to use contain alcohol which helps to dry out the skin and promote healing.

_____ 7. Medicated soaps are a waste of money because the medication washes off when you rinse.

_____ 8. If a product label does not specifically say it has SUGAR in it, then it does not contain sugar.

_____ 9. A good diet for SAFE weight loss is to eat a lot of protein and completely cut out carbohydrates and fats.

_____10. If the ingredients on a can of beef stew are listed as follows: potatoes, peas, carrots, water, spices, and beef, then there is very little beef in the beef stew.

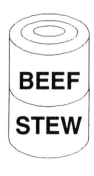

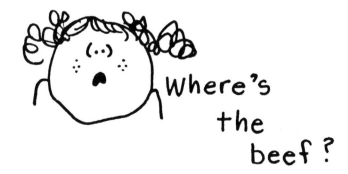

SAFETY

- **Fire Prevention**

- **Poison Prevention**

- **Auto Safety**

- **Bicycle Safety**

- **Water Safety**

- **Environmental Safety**

Name _____ **Date** _____

FIRE PREVENTION CHECKLIST (CH-35)

DIRECTIONS: How safe is your home? Circle YES or NO for each question asked about fire safety. If you can answer YES to all questions, you are doing a good job of preventing fires. If you answered NO to any questions, what can you do to change the situation?

(circle one)

1. Do you have smoke detectors on each floor of your house and outside all bedrooms?   YES   NO

2. Has your family practiced a fire escape plan?   YES   NO

3. Do you have fire extinguishers available in the kitchen, garage, and on all floors of your house?   YES   NO

4. Are electrical sockets NOT overloaded?   YES   NO

5. Are cords in good order (not frayed or cracked)?   YES   NO

6. Are cords in a safe place (NOT under rugs)?   YES   NO

7. Are matches and lighters out of reach of small children?   YES   NO

8. Do you discourage smokers from smoking in bed?   YES   NO

9. Is the pilot light on your gas stove working?   YES   NO

10. Are flammable materials stored away from heat sources?   YES   NO

11. Do you use a cover when cooking oil at high temperatures?   YES   NO

12. Do you store flammable materials in labeled, fireproof containers?   YES   NO

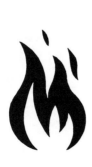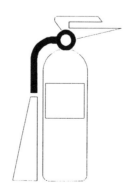

Name _____   **Date** _____

FIRE HOUSE (CH-36)

DIRECTIONS: Listed below are the three components required to have a fire. In the box are examples of fuel, heat sources, and air. Place each word in the box under the correct category. If any one component of a fire is removed, there can be no fire.

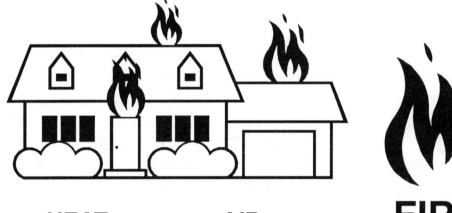

FUEL + **HEAT** + **AIR** = **FIRE**

FUEL:
_____
_____
_____
_____
_____
_____
_____
_____
_____

HEAT:
_____
_____
_____
_____
_____

OXYGEN	GASOLINE
COAL	HEATERS
FIREWORKS	NAIL POLISH REMOVER
FIREPLACE	LIGHTER FLUID
STOVES	CIGARETTES
RAGS	ELECTRICAL WIRES
OIL	PAINT THINNER
KEROSENE	PAPER
MATCHES	RUBBING ALCOHOL
	FURNITURE POLISH

FIRE ESCAPE (CH-37)

DIRECTIONS: For the house plan below, place an asterisk (*) at each point that you think
requires a smoke detector. Next, draw lines indicating an escape route from
each bedroom. Use a different colored line for each route.

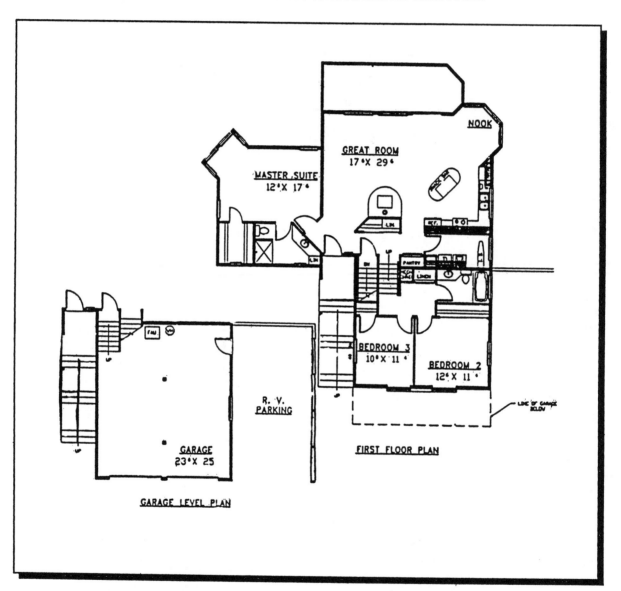

Escape Route --------------------------->
Smoke Detectors (*)

©1993 by The Center for Applied Research in Education

ACTIVITY # 5: POISON PATROL

Concept/ Description: Unsafe storage of medicines and dangerous chemicals is responsible for thousands of poisonings each year.

Objectives: To demonstrate how difficult it is to distinguish between safe and dangerous products. To emphasize how much more difficult this is for young children.

Materials: Cleanser, flour, and powdered sugar in separate plastic bags
Fruit punch, cough syrup, and mouthwash in separate but similar containers
Milk and white paint in similar containers
Ammonia, water, and clear soda in similar containers
Bleach and Mountain Dew® in similar containers
Semi-sweet chocolate and chocolate-flavored laxative
Tic-Tacs®, pills, vitamins, and candies that could be mistaken for medicine and vice-versa
Numbered stick-on labels
POISON PATROL answer sheet (CH-38)

Directions:
1. Label all the products with a number.
2. Place them in an area where you can constantly monitor all the products.
3. Give each student a POISON PATROL answer sheet.
4. Ask students to circle whether they think the product is dangerous (D) or safe (S) and then guess what each product is. DO NOT ALLOW STUDENTS TO TOUCH, SMELL, OR OPEN ANY CONTAINER OR ITEM.
5. Most students will get answers incorrect. Discuss how even one wrong answer could be dangerous. Discuss the implications for small children who put anything and everything in their mouths. Further ask if the students think it's a good idea to make vitamins in the shape of popular cartoon characters. Why or why not?

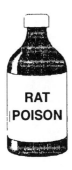

RAT POISON

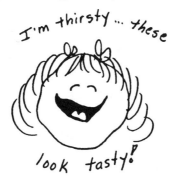

I'm thirsty ... these look tasty!

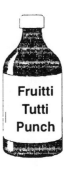

Fruitti Tutti Punch

POISON PATROL Answer Sheet (CH-38)

DIRECTIONS: Look at each item on display. For each numbered item, circle (D) for DANGER-
OUS or (S) for SAFE by the corresponding number. Then, in the blank provided,
try to guess exactly what each item is. DO NOT TOUCH, SMELL, OR OPEN
ANY CONTAINER OR ITEM!

ITEM #	SAFE (S) or DANGEROUS (D) (circle one)			GUESS THE ITEM
1	S	or	D	_____
2	S	or	D	_____
3	S	or	D	_____
4	S	or	D	_____
5	S	or	D	_____
6	S	or	D	_____
7	S	or	D	_____
8	S	or	D	_____
9	S	or	D	_____
10	S	or	D	_____
11	S	or	D	_____
12	S	or	D	_____
13	S	or	D	_____
14	S	or	D	_____
15	S	or	D	_____
16	S	or	D	_____
17	S	or	D	_____
18	S	or	D	_____
19	S	or	D	_____
20	S	or	D	_____

©1993 by The Center for Applied Research in Education

PICK YOUR POISON (CH-39)

DIRECTIONS: Listed below are the descriptions for three types of poisoning: oral, inhalation, and contact. Research the first aid for each type of poisoning and place your answers in the boxes next to each type.

ORAL POISONING

Swallowing a harmful substance, such as bleach, medicines, or poisonous plants.
<u>Signs</u>: sudden, severe stomach pain; nausea or vomiting; burns on or around the mouth; drowsiness; chemical odor on the breath; dilated or constricted pupils; container from a harmful substance nearby.

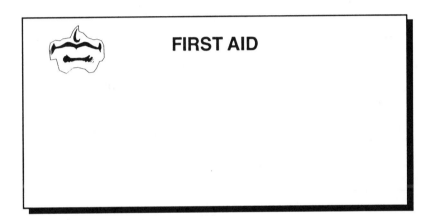

FIRST AID

INHALATION POISONING

Breathing dangerous gases or fumes, such as car exhaust, glue, paints, solvents, and fuels.
<u>Signs</u>: dizziness or headache followed by unconsciousness.

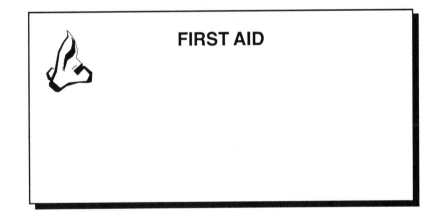

FIRST AID

CONTACT POISONING

Touching a dangerous substance, such as solvents, pesticides, and plants, such as poison ivy, poison oak, and poison sumac.
<u>Signs</u>: rash, swelling, burning, itching, blisters.

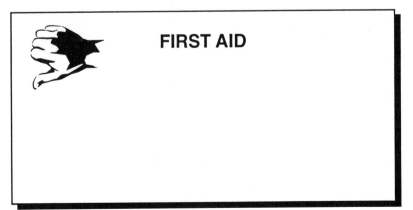

FIRST AID

ON THE LOOKOUT! (CH-40)

DIRECTIONS: Cut out all the articles in the newspaper dealing with auto accidents for two weeks. For each accident, determine if the cause was due to speeding, drinking and driving, poor road conditions, etc., and fill in the chart below. When completed, report your findings to the class.

ACCIDENTS DUE TO:				
Drinking and Driving	**Speeding Conditions**	**Poor Road**	**Other (specify)**	**Were seat belts worn?**

SEAT BELTS *DO* SAVE LIVES (CH-41)

DIRECTIONS: Eighty percent (80%) of all young people killed in automobile accidents last year would still be alive today if they had been wearing a seat belt. Survey your teachers, classmates, friends, family, and neighbors and fill in the chart below. For people who never wear seat belts, ask them why and record their response. Determine the percentage of people you surveyed who wear seat belts all the time. Compare your results with your classmates'.

NAME	AGE	ALWAYS WEAR SEAT BELTS	SOMETIMES WEAR SEAT BELTS	NEVER WEAR SEAT BELTS	RESPONSE
Pat	25			X	Annoying

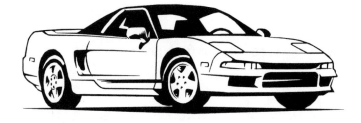

Name _____ Date _____

ARE YOU A SAFE RIDER? (CH-42)

DIRECTIONS: Place a check next to each safety rule YOU observe when riding a bike.

DO YOU...

use crosswalks to walk your bike across busy intersections?_____

always wear a safety helmet?_____

have reflective tape on your bike and clothing?_____

ride single file on the right with the flow of traffic?_____

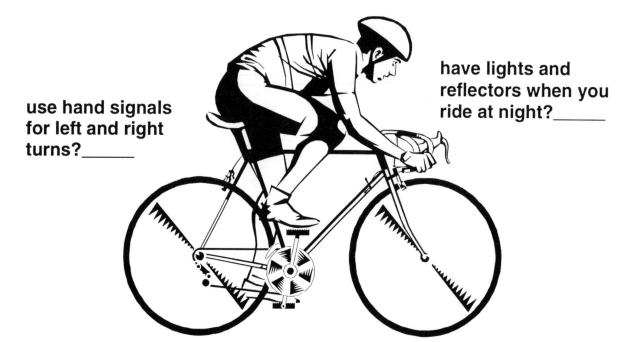

have lights and reflectors when you ride at night?_____

use hand signals for left and right turns?_____

watch for potholes, sewer grates, oil, and other road hazards?_____

use designated bike paths when available?_____

refuse to carry riders on your bike?_____

inspect your bike before each use?_____

BIKE SAFETY SURVEY (CH-43)

DIRECTIONS: Every year nearly 200,000 young people are injured in bicycle-related accidents. Many of these accidents could have been prevented. Survey ten people
who have had a bike accident and record the results below. Discuss your
findings with the class and determine the most common cause of bike accidents.

NAME	ACCIDENT DESCRIPTION (use code below)	APPROX. AGE AT TIME OF ACCIDENT	INJURY SUFFERED
Tony Smith	(2) His shoe laces got caught in the spokes.	14	Dislocated shoulder.

ACCIDENT DESCRIPTION CODE:

1 = The accident was due to a loss of control.
2 = Clothing became entangled in the bike.
3 = There was a collision with another bike, car, etc.
4 = A foot slipped off the pedal.
5 = There was a mechanical problem with the bicycle.

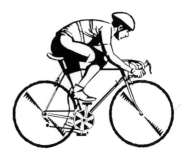

WATER SAFETY UNSCRAMBLE (CH-44)

DIRECTIONS: Unscramble the jumbled words to reveal ten water safety rules. Place the unscrambled word in the blank to the right.

1. Don't swim immediately after taegni.   _____

2. Always swim in an area where a filedgrua is present.   _____

3. Always swim with a dduby.   _____

4. Don't use underwater equipment unless you have been raintde.   _____

5. Wear a lotfaatoin device when required.   _____

6. Never dive in an desnspvuueri or unfamiliar area.   _____

7. Never swim or dive after using laocohl or other drugs.   _____

8. Do not walk on cie that may be unsafe.   _____

9. If you are on ice that begins to crack, lie down and rwcal to shore.   _____

10. Learn poofdrrwongin techniques.   _____

ACTIVITY 6: ENVIRONMENTAL HAZARDS

Concept/ Description: There are many types of catastrophic events that may be natural disasters, the result of technology, or caused by human error. We should be aware of these hazards and prepare ourselves whenever possible.

Objective: To make a mural of environmental hazards and their devastating effects and to research precautions and safety rules for each.

Materials: Large roll of brown paper or butcher paper
Colored markers, pens, crayons, or paint and brushes
Magazine or newspaper articles about natural and man-made disasters
Reference books about natural and man-made disasters

Directions: 1. Divide the class into groups of four or five.

2. Give each group a large sheet of brown paper and some drawing materials.

3. Ask some groups to draw murals depicting *natural disasters* and their effects on the environment. Disasters could include:

   - hurricanes
   - tornadoes
   - floods
   - earthquakes
   - blizzards

4. Ask other groups to draw murals depicting *man-made disasters* and their effects on the environment. Disasters could include:

   - nuclear power plant accidents
   - forest fires (unless caused by lightning)
   - illegal dumping of toxic wastes
   - hazardous material spills
   - air pollution, toxic fumes

5. Assign each group a topic to research and have them report back to the class. Reports should include safety procedures and precautions as well as examples of the type of disaster and the appropriate response.

ACTIVITY 7: IT'S HAZARDOUS TO YOUR HEALTH

Concept/ Description: There are many types of environmental hazards. We should be aware of these and prepare ourselves whenever possible.

Objective: To collect magazine and newspaper articles dealing with environmental hazards and construct a bulletin board.

Materials: Bulletin board
Newspaper and magazine articles dealing with environmental hazards
Staples and stapler
Construction paper

Directions:
1. Divide a bulletin board into two sections and, using cut-out letters, label one section *Man-Made Hazards* and the other *Natural Hazards*.

2. As the school year progresses, ask students to cut out and bring to class articles dealing with environmental hazards. Determine if the hazard was a result of nature or caused by humans. Place the article in the proper section on the bulletin board.

3. Man-made hazards include: nuclear power plant accidents, hazardous material spills, illegal dumping of toxic wastes, forest or brush fires (unless caused by lightning).

   Natural hazards include: floods, tornadoes, earthquakes, blizzards, and hurricanes.

4. At the end of the year, determine if there was more damage to the environment caused by humans or by nature. Discuss ways we can keep our environment safe.

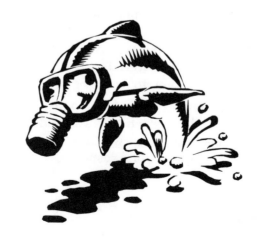

ACCIDENTS

- **Causes of Accidents**

- **Safety Rules**

I'VE FALLEN AND I CAN'T GET UP! (CH-45)

DIRECTIONS: For each box below, list THREE (3) ways that a person could get hurt.

In the kitchen...

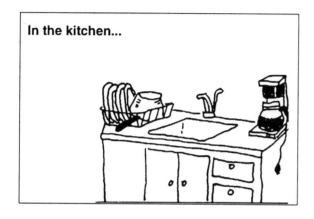

In the bathroom...

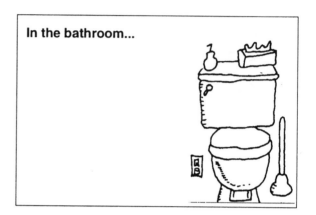

In school...

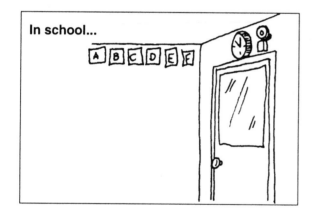

At the pool...

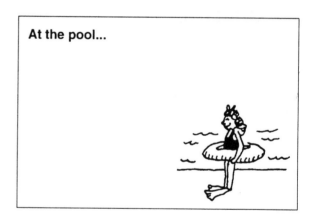

In the neighborhood...

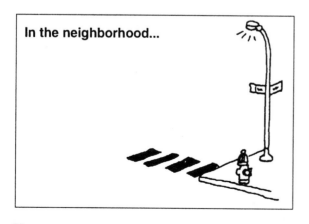

On the job...

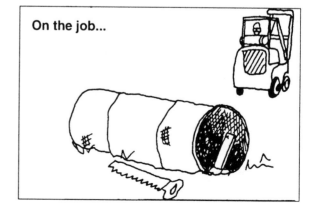

Name _____ **Date** _____

IT WAS AN ACCIDENT! (CH-46)

DIRECTIONS: Look at the chart below that deals with the leading causes of accidental death, then answer the questions.

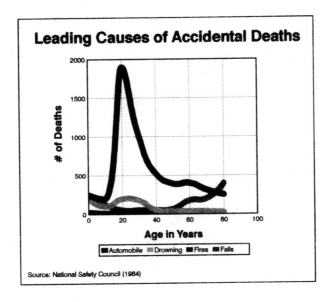

Leading Causes of Accidental Deaths

# of Deaths / Age in Years

Automobile Drowning Fires Falls

Source: National Safety Council (1984)

1. According to the chart, which age group suffered the most deaths from auto accidents?

_____

2. Why do you think this is the case? _____

_____

3. Which age group is most susceptible to death from falls? _____

4. Why do you think this is the case? _____

_____

5. Which two age groups seem to have the most deaths from drowning?

_____

6. Give some reasons for this. _____

_____

Name _____ **Date** _____

THERE'S NO PLACE LIKE HOME (CH-47)

DIRECTIONS: Look at the chart below that deals with the leading causes of accidental deaths in the home, then answer the questions.

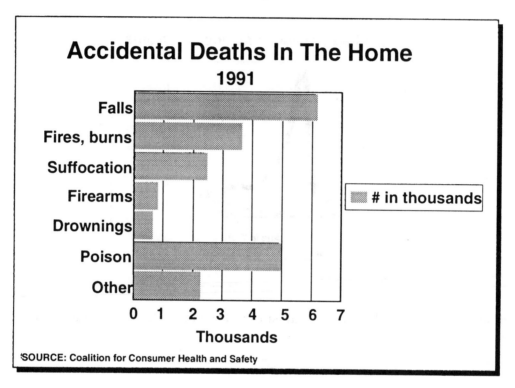

1. According to the chart, what is the leading cause of accidental death in the home?

_____

2. What could be done to eliminate this hazard? _____

3. What is the second leading cause of accidental home deaths? _____

4. What age group do you think is most affected by this?_____

   Why? _____

5. Give examples of what you think the "other" category might include:

_____

_____

Name _____ **Date** _____

BE CAREFUL, YOU'LL POKE YOUR EYE OUT! (CH-48)

DIRECTIONS: List all the safety rules that you can recall from your childhood. List the possible consequences of NOT following that particular rule and put an asterisk (*) next to any consequences you, personally, suffered.

SAFETY RULES	POSSIBLE CONSEQUENCES
Don't jump on the beds.	Broken bones, concussion (*), cuts, bruises(*)

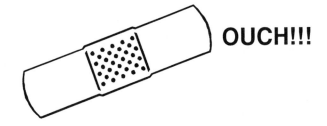 **OUCH!!!**

AN OUNCE OF PREVENTION (CH-49)

DIRECTIONS: For each box below, list **THREE (3)** safety rules that should be followed in order to prevent an accident.

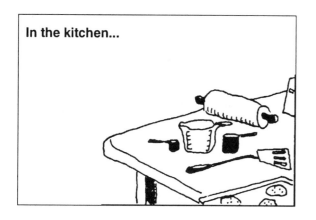

In the kitchen...

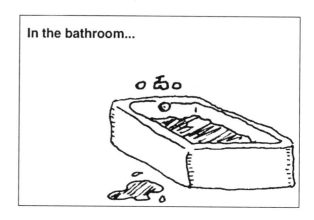

In the bathroom...

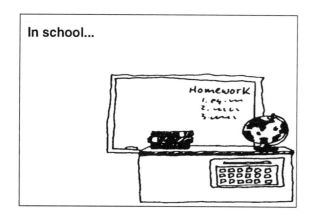

In school...

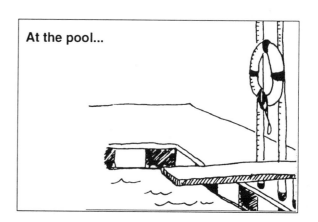

At the pool...

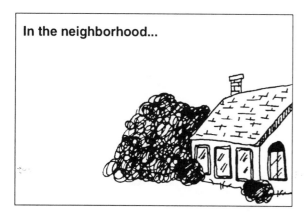

In the neighborhood...

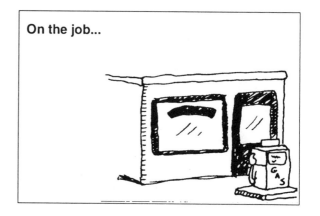

On the job...

ACTIVITY 8: WHEEL OF ADVERSITY

Concept/ Description: Students will attempt to win the game by correctly answering questions about first aid and safety.

Objective: To be the first group to cross the finish line and be declared the winner

Materials: WHEEL OF ADVERSITY Game Wheel (CH-50)
WHEEL OF ADVERSITY Desk Signs (CH 51-52)
WHEEL OF ADVERSITY Question Cards (CH 53-55)
Four differently colored pinnies (or squares of construction paper)
Chairs (or desks) arranged as shown in figure 1
Tape
One die
ACCIDENT Cards (CH 56-57)

Directions:

1. Arrange the desks or chairs as shown. If this is not possible, use the floor tiles as squares. The classroom is the gameboard and designated students will move from chair to chair (or tile to tile).

2. Prior to class, photocopy the desk signs so that you have one HOSPITAL and one DOCTOR'S OFFICE sign and ten ACCIDENT signs. Tape the HOSPITAL sign somewhere in the first row and the DOCTOR'S OFFICE sign somewhere in the second row. Place the ACCIDENT signs randomly on any ten chairs or desks.

3. Separate the cards into categories. (You may wish to write the categories on the back of each card.)

4. Divide the class into four groups and assign each group a color according to the color of the pinnies or construction paper you have. Ask one member of each group to be the "playing piece" and wear the pinnie (or tape the construction paper to his or her back). That person will physically move from chair to chair as if moving over a gameboard.

5. To start the game, one person from the RED team (for example) would spin the wheel. If the spinner landed on the category "First Aid," the teacher would ask the group a question on first aid. If the group answers correctly, it's their turn to roll the die and the person wearing the pinnie moves the corresponding number of chairs. If the answer is incorrect, the group does not roll the die and just remains as is.

6. If a student lands on an ACCIDENT SQUARE, the group chooses an ACCIDENT CARD and follows the directions.

7. Play proceeds from group to group, and the first group to have its person reach the last chair is the winner.

Figure 1. Classroom Setup for Wheel of Adversity

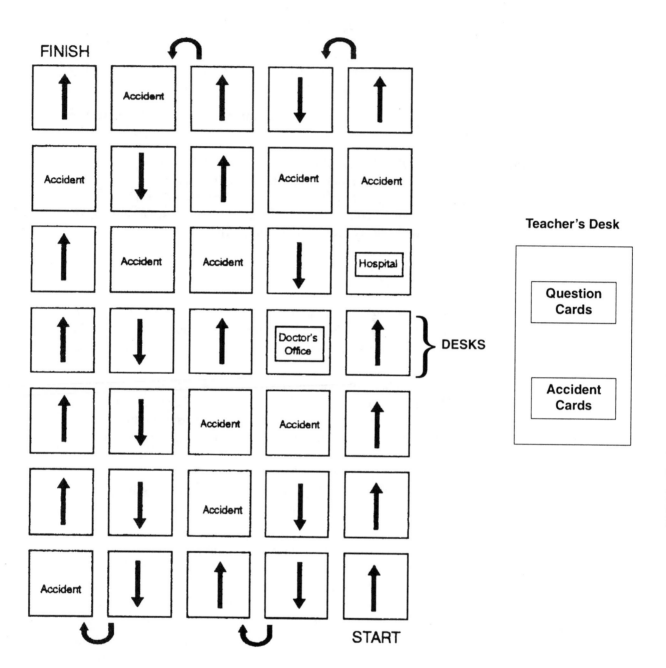

Red Team	Blue Team	Yellow Team	Green Team
X X	X X	X X	X X
XX	XX	XX	XX
X X	X X	X X	X X
X	X	X	X

WHEEL OF ADVERSITY Game Wheel (CH-50)

DIRECTIONS: Cut out the base and glue to oaktag or laminate. Trace the spinner onto oaktag and cut it out. Attach the spinner to the base by placing a paper fastener through the center of the wheel and the spinner. Be sure to fasten loosely so it can spin. Mark one end of the spinner with marker to indicate which end of the spinner is pointing to the category.

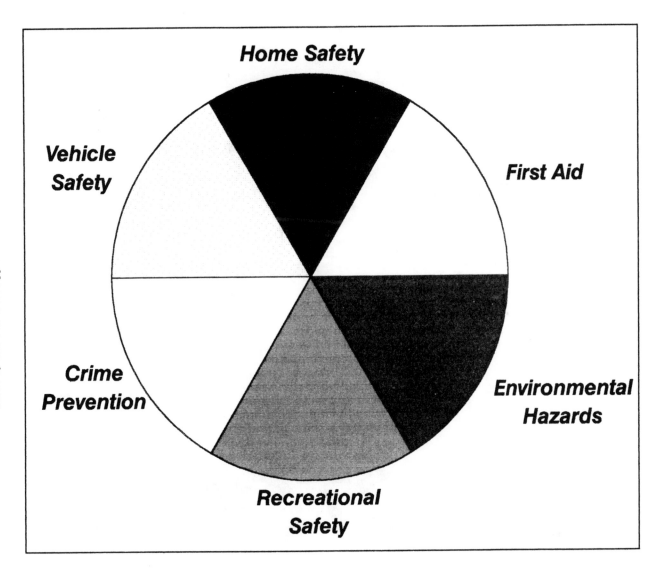

SPINNER (Trace onto oaktag and cut.):

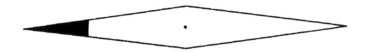

DIRECTIONS: Cut out the signs and place on two desks as explained in the game directions.

HOSPITAL

DOCTOR'S OFFICE

WHEEL OF ADVERSITY Desk Signs (CH-52)

DIRECTIONS: Make five copies of this sheet, cut out the signs, and place them on ten desks as explained in the game directions.

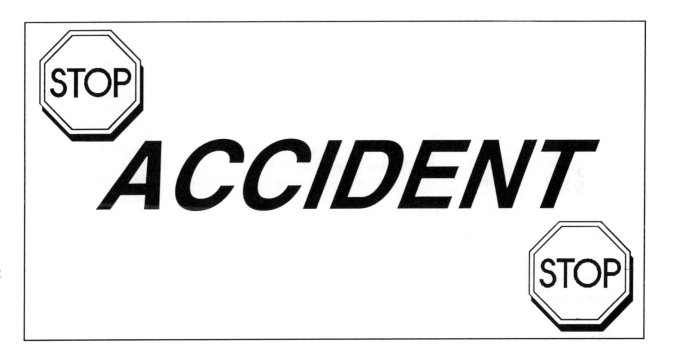

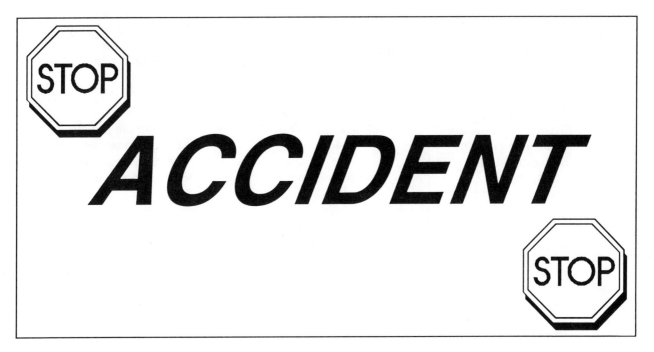

WHEEL OF ADVERSITY Question Cards (CH-53)

Home Safety What age group is most likely to be injured in falls? (Children and the elderly)	**Home Safety** Where do 1/3 of all accidents occur? (In the home)	**Home Safety** What is the leading cause of death from home accidents? (Falls)
Home Safety Name a common cause of household fires. (Smoking, wiring, kids playing with matches, improper storage)	**Home Safety** If your clothing catches fire, what should you do? (Stop, drop, roll)	**Home Safety** What is syrup of ipecac used for? (Accidental poisoning to induce vomiting)
Home Safety What is death from exposure to electricity called? (Electrocution)	**Home Safety** Where should you call in case of accidental poisoning? (Poison Control Center)	**Home Safety** To avoid electrocution, where should you never use appliances? (Near water)
Vehicle Safety Over 50% of all auto accidents have been linked to what? (Alcohol)	**Vehicle Safety** What auto safety device must be worn in many states? (Seat belts)	**Vehicle Safety** Show the proper bike signal for a left turn. (Left arm straight out at shoulder height)
Vehicle Safety What should always be worn when riding a bike or motorcycle? (A helmet)	**Vehicle Safety** On which side of the road should you ride a bike? (With the flow of traffic on the right side of the road)	**Vehicle Safety** Where do most bicycle accidents occur? (At intersections)
Vehicle Safety While driving on a slippery road, should you use the brake or shift to a lower gear? (Shift to a lower gear)	**Vehicle Safety** Which age group has the most auto accidents: 15–24, 25–34, or 35 and over? (15–24)	**Vehicle Safety** What is the leading cause of accidental death? (Auto accidents)
Crime Prevention What is the crime in which a person is forced to have sexual relations? (Rape)	**Crime Prevention** What should you never let a caller know? (That you are alone)	**Crime Prevention** If a person tries to steal your wallet at gunpoint, what should you do? (Give them the wallet)

WHEEL OF ADVERSITY Question Cards (CH-54)

Crime Prevention If your car breaks down, should you get out of the car or remain inside? (Remain inside)	**Crime Prevention** If raped, what should the victim do immediately? (Seek medical attention and call the police)	**Crime Prevention** Rapes are usually committed by someone the victim knows: True or False? (True)
Crime Prevention If a car drives next to you while you are walking, what should you do? (Quickly walk in the opposite direction)	**Crime Prevention** Where should you not hide keys? (Under a doormat, in the mailbox, above the door)	**Crime Prevention** What should you avoid while walking? (Deserted places, dark areas, doorways, hedges)
Recreational Safety What is the lifesaving method that allows you to float and breathe wthout much energy? (Drownproofing)	**Recreational Safety** What should you do if on ice that begins to crack? (Lie down and crawl to shore)	**Recreational Safety** What piece of safety equipment should every person in a boat wear? (A life jacket)
Recreational Safety How should you remove a stinger from a bee sting? (Scrape across it with your nail or cardboard)	**Recreational Safety** Why is it dangerous to dive into unknown water? (Possibility of neck injury)	**Recreational Safety** Name a poisonous plant you might encounter when camping. (Poison oak, ivy, or sumac)
Recreational Safety What should you do if you sprain your ankle while jogging? (Apply ice, compression, and elevation)	**Recreational Safety** If you experience frostbite, should you massage the area, or immerse it in warm water? (Immerse in warm water)	**Recreational Safety** If a person suffers from heat stroke, do they perspire? (No)
Environmental Hazards If caught outdoors during a tornado, how should you run? (At right angles to its path)	**Environmental Hazards** If you are driving during an earthquake, what should you do? (Pull over and stop)	**Environmental Hazards** What type of storm is characterized by heavy rains and winds over 75 mph? (A hurricane)
Environmental Hazards How much water should you store in case of a disaster? (A two-week supply)	**Environmental Hazards** During what emergency should you stand in an interior doorway? (An earthquake)	**Environmental Hazards** Name a man-made disaster. (Nuclear accident, oil spill, illegal dumping of toxic wastes, some forest fires)

WHEEL OF ADVERSITY Question Cards (CH-55)

Environmental Hazards What does an earthquake on the ocean floor cause? (Tidal waves or tsunami)	**Environmental Hazards** During what emergency should you get to high ground? (Flood)	**Environmental Hazards** What does a flood warning mean? (Flooding will occur)
First Aid What should you not do if you suspect neck or spinal injury? (Move the victim)	**First Aid** Which is an early sign of shock: pale, clammy skin or dry, red skin? (Pale, clammy skin)	**First Aid** What is the name of the procedure that uses external heart massage and rescue breathing? (CPR)
First Aid Show the international signal for choking. (Hand across throat)	**First Aid** What should you apply to a first-degree burn? (Cold water)	**First Aid** For which condition would you have a person breathe into a paper bag? (Hyperventilation)

WHEEL OF ADVERSITY Accident Cards (CH-56)

**You fell off your skateboard and you weren't wearing pads.
GO BACK 2 SPACES**

**You forgot to check your bike and the chain fell off, causing you to fall.
GO BACK 3 SPACES**

**You saved a drowning victim.
GO AHEAD 5 SPACES**

**You were stung by a bee.
GO BACK 1 SPACE**

**While babysitting, you recognized the signs of oral poisoning and called the Poison Control Center.
GO AHEAD 3 SPACES**

**You were fooling around and fractured your ankle.
GO TO THE HOSPITAL**

**FREE CARD
Hold this card and turn it in whenever you want to ignore the instructions on an
ACCIDENT CARD**

**You got in a fight and your nose is bleeding.
GO BACK 1 SPACE**

WHEEL OF ADVERSITY Accident Cards (CH-57)

You didn't wear your seat belt. **GO BACK 3 SPACES**	You successfully performed the Heimlich Maneuver and saved a life. **GO AHEAD 5 SPACES**
You drove under the influence of alcohol and had an auto accident. **GO TO THE HOSPITAL AND LOSE 1 TURN**	You swam in an area without a lifeguard. **GO BACK 2 SPACES**
You passed your Red Cross CPR class. **GO AHEAD 4 SPACES**	You stepped on a nail and need a tetanus shot. **GO TO THE DOCTOR'S OFFICE**
You treated a victim for heart attack. **ROLL AGAIN AND MOVE THE NUMBER OF SPACES ON THE DIE**	You burned yourself playing with matches. **GO TO THE HOSPITAL**

Name _____ **Date** _____

WHAT'S WRONG WITH THIS PICTURE? (CH-58)

DIRECTIONS: On the back of this sheet, list everything wrong with each picture.

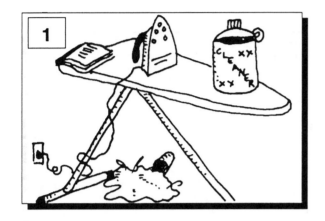

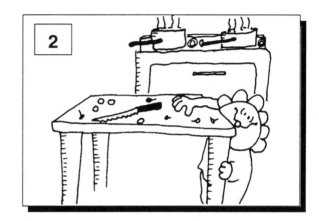

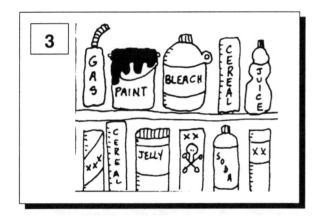

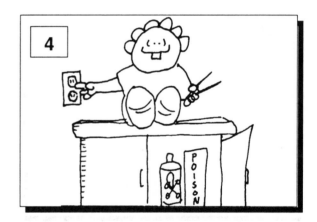

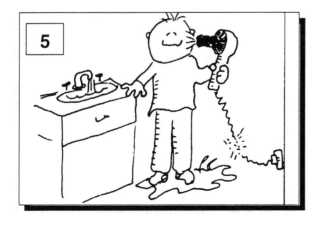

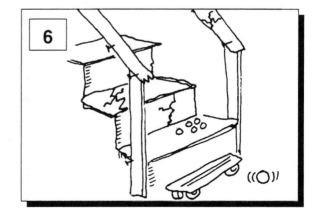

Name ______________________________ Date ______________

WHAT'S WRONG WITH THIS PICTURE? (2) (CH-59)

DIRECTIONS: Design your own scenes showing unsafe behaviors. When completed, exchange papers with a classmate and circle the unsafe behaviors. Discuss.

1

2

3

4

5

6

ACTIVITY 9: KNOW THE RULES

Concept/
Description: Students should know and follow appropriate safety practices for many different situations.

Objective: To fill in correct safety and emergency procedures and be the first to reach the finish line.

Materials: One "KNOW THE RULES" GAMEBOARD per student (CH-60)
One set of "KNOW THE RULES" game cards per group of four students (CH 61-63)
Pens or pencils
Timer or stopwatch

Directions: 1. Cut the game cards and separate.

2. Divide the class into groups of four and give each group a set of game cards placed face down.

3. Give each student a gameboard.

4. On the teacher's signal, ask each group member to choose ONE card, read it silently, and quickly list all the safety rules he or she can think of for that situation in the squares on the gameboard. List one rule or practice per square. For example, if the card "AUTO SAFETY" was chosen, the student could write "wear seat belts, don't drink and drive, observe the speed limits, observe traffic signals," and thereby move four spaces on the board. The teacher can set a time limit of 15 seconds, 30 seconds, etc., depending on the age of the group. When time is up, announce that they are to pick a new card and proceed with play.

5. Continue until someone in the class reaches the end square.

6. Go back over the cards and discuss the rules and procedures as a class.

Variations: 1. To make the game competitive among the groups, continue until one group of four has reached the end and declare that group the winner.

2. Use one gameboard per group and have a "secretary" record the group's responses.

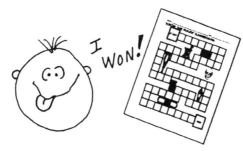

"KNOW THE RULES" GAMEBOARD (CH-60)

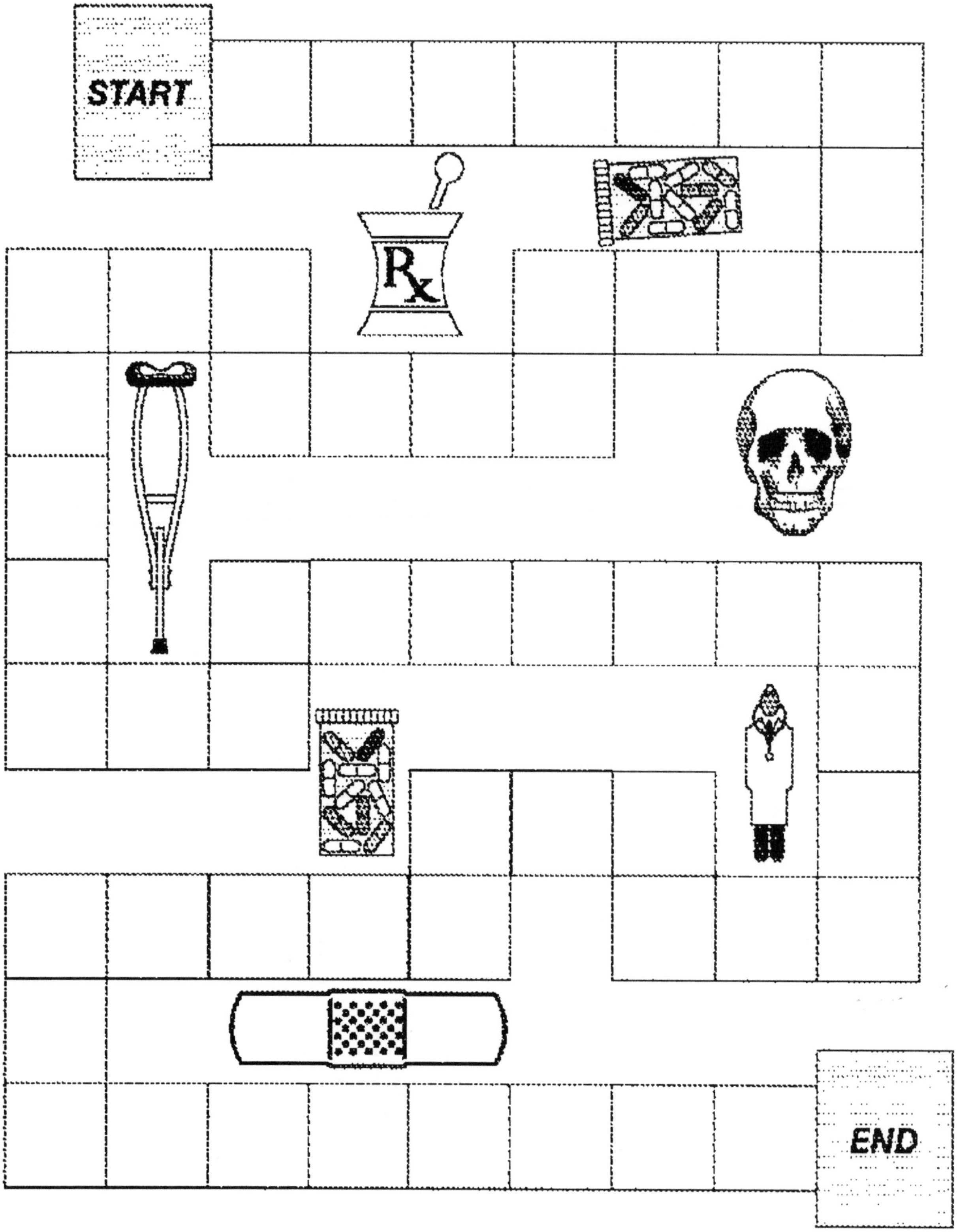

©1993 by The Center for Applied Research in Education

START

END

"KNOW THE RULES" Game Cards (CH-61)

BICYCLING	AUTO SAFETY
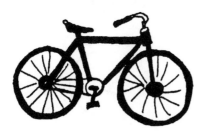	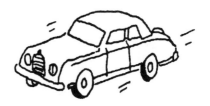
FOOTBALL	**SKATEBOARDING OR SKATING**
	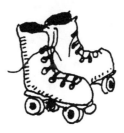
LIGHTNING	**SWIMMING**
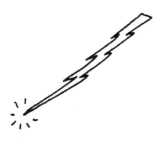	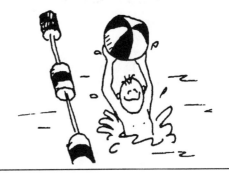
BABYSITTING	**STORING POISONS**
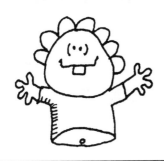	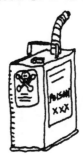

"KNOW THE RULES" Game Cards (CH-62)

EXPOSURE TO EXTREME COLD 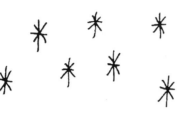	**EXPOSURE TO EXTREME HEAT** 
BLEEDING 	**CHOKING** 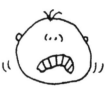
ANIMAL BITES 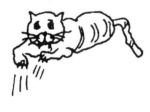	**INSECT STINGS**
RESCUE BREATHING 	**BROKEN BONES** 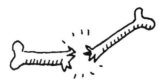

"KNOW THE RULES" Game Cards (CH-63)

TORNADO	EARTHQUAKE
SOCCER, HOCKEY, OR LACROSSE	**STRANGERS**
ELECTRICITY	**HOUSE FIRES**
COOKING	**EXPOSURE TO SUN**

MAKE YOUR OWN Game Cards (CH-64)

SAFETY TOONS (CH-65)

DIRECTIONS: In the boxes below, design your own safety comic strips. Each strip must include at least one safety rule.

SAFETY COMIC STRIP 1

SAFETY COMIC STRIP 2

ACTIVITY 10: SLAMMA JAMMA

Concept/ Description: Many situations require knowledge of basic safety rules.

Objective: To score the most points by correctly stating safety rules and shooting baskets.

Materials: SLAMMA JAMMA Cards (CH-66)
Official paper wad (crumpled paper wrapped in masking tape)
Small bucket or trash can (or use one of the popular mini basketball hoops that hang over doors or attach to trashcans)
SLAMMA JAMMA Checklist (CH-67)
Masking tape
Chalkboard and chalk

Directions:

1. Prior to class, cut out the SLAMMA JAMMA Cards and make a copy of the SLAMMA JAMMA Checklist.

2. Divide the class into two equal teams.

3. Place a taped "foul line" on the floor approximately 15 feet from the basket (adjust depending on the age of the group).

4. Lay the SLAMMA JAMMA Cards face down on the teacher's desk.

5. Have one student from Team A pick a card and read it aloud.

6. Anyone from Team A may raise his or her hand and give a safety rule that deals with that topic. If correct, the team is awarded 1 point, plus the person who answered may take one "foul shot." If the foul shot goes in, an additional point is added. If it is missed, the team still retains the point for the correct answer. Play then proceeds to Team B. Score is kept on the chalkboard.

7. After a card is chosen, it is placed back on the table, face down, and the cards are reshuffled. The same card may be picked any number of times. It will become increasingly difficult to list safety rules, however, the more often the card is chosen.

8. If a team cannot give a safety rule or gives an incorrect rule, the opposing team gets a chance to answer and, if correct, shoot. They still get their normal turn and, in effect, would get two turns in a row.

9. The team with more points at the end of the time limit is the winner.

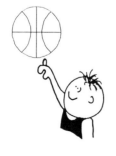

10. The SLAMMA JAMMA Checklist can be used for general reference and for checking off each safety rule as it is mentioned to avoid repeating rules. Extra numbers and space allow you to add other rules.

SLAMMA JAMMA Cards (CH-66)

FALLS

FIRES

BURNS

POISONING

DROWNING

FIREARMS

EARTHQUAKES

TORNADOS

CHOKING
OR
SUFFOCATION

ELECTROCUTION

SLAMMA JAMMA Checklist (CH-67)

FALLS

_____ 1. Keep objects off steps.

_____ 2. Keep objects out of walkways.

_____ 3. Never leave a baby on a raised surface unattended.

_____ 4. Use safety gates with toddlers.

_____ 5. Keep children away from open doors and windows.

_____ 6.

_____ 7.

_____ 8.

FIRES

_____ 1. Install smoke detectors.

_____ 2. Practice a fire escape plan.

_____ 3. Have fire extinguishers.

_____ 4. Keep matches and lighters away from small children.

_____ 5. Avoid careless smoking.

_____ 6. Store flammable liquids away from heat.

_____ 7. Don't overload electrical sockets.

_____ 8. Be sure electrical cords are not frayed or cracked.

_____ 9. Don't place cords under rugs.

_____ 10.

BURNS

_____ 1. Turn pot handles towards the center of the stove.

_____ 2. Test the water in the shower or tub before getting in.

_____ 3. Never use water on a grease fire.

_____ 4. Keep children away from fireplaces, electric heaters, etc.

_____ 5. Don't play with matches.

_____ 6. Don't leave cigarettes unattended.

_____ 7.

_____ 8.

POISONING

_____ 1. Don't leave medicines or poisons within a child's reach.

_____ 2. Clearly label poisonous substances.

_____ 3. Never put poisons in food containers.

_____ 4. Lock up hazardous substances.

_____ 5. Have the poison control center's number handy.

_____ 6. Use products with harmful fumes outdoors or in a ventilated area.

_____ 7.

_____ 8.

ELECTROCUTION

_____ 1. Never try to repair an electrical appliance when it is plugged in.

_____ 2. Keep young children away from electrical outlets.

_____ 3. Never use appliances when you are wet or near water.

_____ 4. Don't use the phone, water, or electrical appliances during a thunderstorm.

_____ 5.

DROWNING

_____ 1. Never swim alone.

_____ 2. Never leave a child alone in the bathroom or near a pool.

_____ 3. Don't swim while under the influence of alcohol or other drugs.

_____ 4. Don't dive in shallow or unknown water.

_____ 5. Follow posted pool rules.

_____ 6.

_____ 7.

_____ 8.

FIREARMS

_____ 1. Keep firearms unloaded and locked up.

_____ 2. Lock ammunition in a separate place.

_____ 3. Always point firearms away from yourself and others when cleaning them.

_____ 4. Do not use firearms unless properly trained.

_____ 5.

_____ 6.

EARTHQUAKES

_____ 1. If inside, brace yourself in an interior doorway or under a table.

_____ 2. Stay away from windows and glass doors.

_____ 3. If outside, stay in an open area, away from walls and buildings.

_____ 4. Stay away from downed electrical lines.

_____ 5. If driving, pull over and stop.

_____ 6.

_____ 7.

TORNADOS

_____ 1. If caught outdoors, move away at right angles to the tornado's path.

_____ 2. Lie flat in the nearest ditch or ravine.

_____ 3. If indoors, go to the lowest floor of the house.

_____ 4. Leave some windows open to equalize pressure, but stay clear of them.

_____ 5. Get out of mobile homes.

_____ 6.

_____ 7.

CHOKING OR SUFFOCATION

_____ 1. Don't run or jump while eating.

_____ 2. Keep small objects out of the reach of children.

_____ 3. Keep plastic bags away from children.

_____ 4. Be sure pillows and bedclothes do not interfere with an infant's breathing.

_____ 5.

_____ 6.

FIRST AID

- **Animals and Insects**

- **Emergency Procedures**

- **General Knowledge**

BITES AND STINGS (CH-68)

DIRECTIONS: Match the insect or animal to the type of treatment, by placing the letter in the box surrounding each picture. Letters may be used more than once.

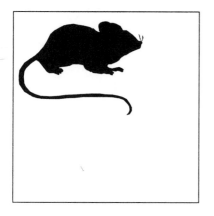

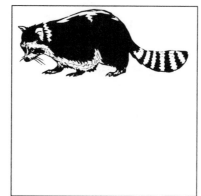

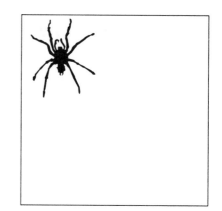

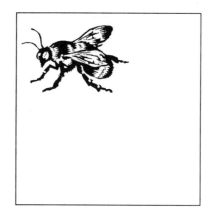

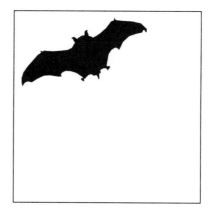

A. Scrape off the stinger with your fingernail, a flat piece of cardboard, or a credit card.

B. Apply ice or a paste of baking soda and water.

C. Keep the victim calm.

D. Wash with soap and water.

E. Seek immediate medical attention and treat for shock.

F. If possible, catch the animal so it can be examined for rabies. Don't risk your health to do so, however.

G. Seek medical attention and notify the health department.

H. Cover the wound with a clean, dry dressing.

Name _____   **Date** _____

BEE SAFE (CH-69)

DIRECTIONS: In the beehive, find and circle the words that explain the symptoms and signs of an allergic reaction to bee stings. Use the clues below to figure out the words.

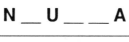

SIGNS AND SYMPTOMS (Clues)

P__ __ __

SHORTNESS OF __ RE__ __ __

__ __DN__ __ __

__ W __ __ __ I __ G

__ __ ZZ __ __ __ __ __

N __ U __ __ A

ACTIVITY 11: RESCUE 911

**Concept/
Description:** There are many trained volunteers in the medical field.

Objectives: To become aware of the job of rescue personnel. To learn some emergency procedures they can follow.

Materials: None

Directions:
1. Contact the local rescue squad and invite a member to speak to your class.
2. Ask the rescue squad member(s) to talk about various situations where they had to administer first aid.
3. Ask them to demonstrate several first aid techniques that a typical teenager could use.
4. Ask them what is the most frequent type of accident they encounter in your area.
5. Ask them to recommend a few safety precautions that your students could take to reduce their risk of injury.

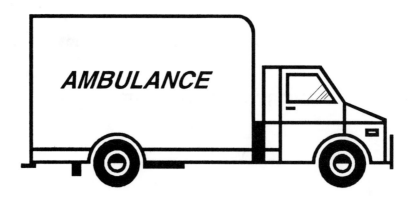

THIS IS AN EMERGENCY!! (CH-70)

DIRECTIONS: Listed below is the information you should give when calling to report an emergency. Look in the local phone book, then write down the numbers.

AMBULANCE _____

POLICE _____

FIRE_____

DOCTOR _____

FATHER'S WORK_____

MOTHER'S WORK _____

POISON CONTROL CENTER _____

NEIGHBOR _____

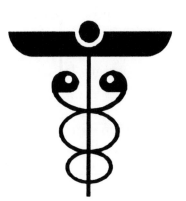

WHEN YOU CALL:

1. Say "THIS IS AN EMERGENCY."
2. Calmly and clearly state the problem.
3. Tell how many people need assistance.
4. Explain the condition of the victim(s).
5. Tell what is currently being done to help.
6. Give your address and directions, if needed.
7. Give your telephone number.
8. STAY ON THE LINE UNTIL THE PERSON TO WHOM YOU ARE SPEAKING HANGS UP.

Name _____ Date _____

BE A LIFESAVER! (CH-71)

DIRECTIONS: Using the words in the box, fill in the steps you should take to help someone who may be experiencing a life or death situation.

DRIVE	PULSE
EMERGENCY	QUIETLY
LICENSED	BREATHING
911	TRAINED
CPR	SPEAK
INTERFERE	HEIMLICH

1. If you are with someone who is having a heart attack or stroke, have him or her rest_____.

2. Call the_____medical system (EMS). This could be the fire department, an ambulance service,_____, or other emergency number.

3. If driving the victim to the hospital would be faster, then a_____ driver should take the victim there. Do not let the victim_____.

4. If the person has no_____or is not_____, perform_____if you are_____.

5. If the person is choking and can_____, breathe, or cough do not _____unless his or her condition gets worse.

6. If the victim is choking and cannot breathe or speak, perform the_____ Maneuver if you are trained to do so.

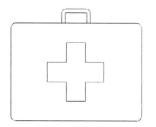

HELP!!!!

SPLIT-SECOND DECISION (CH-72)

DIRECTIONS: For each situation, list the steps you should take when faced with that emergency. Use the SPLIT-SECOND DECISION Worksheet (CH-73).

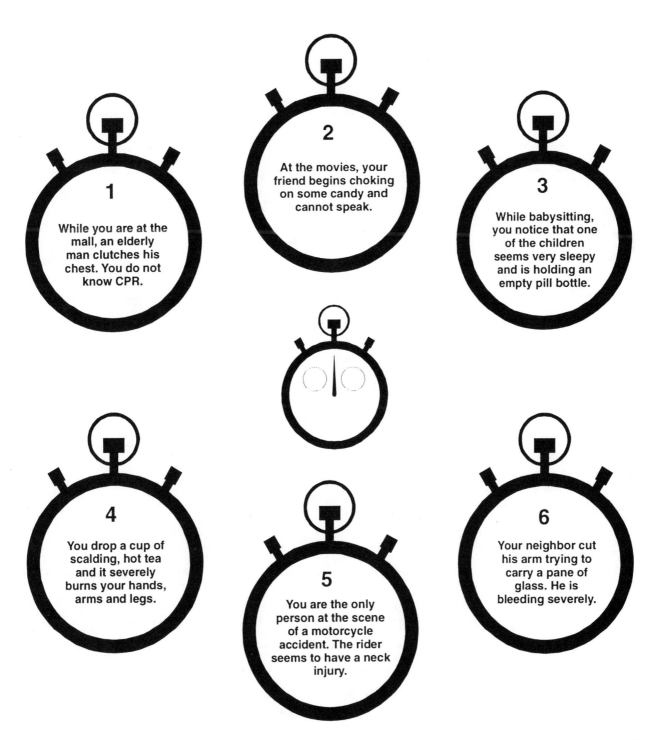

1 While you are at the mall, an elderly man clutches his chest. You do not know CPR.

2 At the movies, your friend begins choking on some candy and cannot speak.

3 While babysitting, you notice that one of the children seems very sleepy and is holding an empty pill bottle.

4 You drop a cup of scalding, hot tea and it severely burns your hands, arms and legs.

5 You are the only person at the scene of a motorcycle accident. The rider seems to have a neck injury.

6 Your neighbor cut his arm trying to carry a pane of glass. He is bleeding severely.

SPLIT-SECOND DECISION Worksheet (CH-73)

① 1

_____

_____

_____

_____

_____

_____

② 2

_____

_____

_____

_____

_____

_____

③ 3

_____

_____

_____

_____

_____

_____

_____

④ 4

_____

_____

_____

_____

_____

_____

_____

⑤ 5

_____

_____

_____

_____

_____

_____

_____

⑥ 6

_____

_____

_____

_____

_____

_____

_____

TEST YOUR FIRST AID I.Q. (CH-74)

DIRECTIONS: Place the letter of the best answer in the blank to the left.

_____ 1. After you have rescued a person, the FIRST thing you should do is
     a. get help.
     b. check the victim's breathing.
     c. control severe bleeding.

_____ 2. Which is not a preferred way to control bleeding?
     a. Apply direct pressure to the wound.
     b. Use pressure points.
     c. Apply a tourniquet.

_____ 3. Which is NOT a sign of shock?
     a. Shallow, uneven breathing.
     b. The skin is dry, warm, and reddish.
     c. The pulse is weak or cannot be felt.

_____ 4. Which is NOT a method of helping a poisoning victim?
     a. Call a poison control center or a doctor and follow instructions.
     b. Save the container of the poisonous substance and show it to the medical team when they arrive.
     c. Immediately induce vomiting.

_____ 5. Which SHOULD be done in case of a third-degree burn?
     a. Cover the burned area with a clean dressing.
     b. Remove burned clothing.
     c. Apply ice to the burn.

_____ 6. If you are stung by a wasp or bee, you should
     a. pull out the stinger with a pair of tweezers.
     b. scrape across the stinger with a piece of cardboard or credit card.
     c. leave the stinger alone and apply ice.

_____ 7. If a person suffers a sprained ankle, you should
     a. raise the sprained part and apply heat.
     b. lower the sprained part and apply ice.
     c. raise the sprained part and apply cold packs.

_____ 8. First aid for a nosebleed is
     a. sit, lean forward, and pinch the nose firmly for 5 minutes.
     b. lie down and pinch the nose shut for 5 minutes.
     c. tilt the head back and apply ice to the back of the neck.

_____ 9. If a person faints, you should
     a. pour water over his or her face.
     b. raise his or her legs 8 to 12 inches.
     c. try to help him or her to a standing position.

_____ 10. The Good Samaritan Law says that anyone who tries to help in an emergency
     a. must be certified in first aid.
     b. cannot be sued unless he or she knowingly acted unsafely.

EMERGENCY TERMS YOU SHOULD KNOW (CH-75)

DIRECTIONS: Review the words below, then find them in the Seek and Find. Words may be vertical, horizontal, or diagonal, frontwards and backwards.

CPR (Cardiopulmonary Resuscitation)—A technique in which breathing is restored by mouth-to-mouth resuscitation and heartbeat is restored by chest compression.

HEIMLICH MANEUVER—A method of helping a choking victim by performing under-the-diaphragm abdominal thrusts to expel an object blocking the trachea (windpipe).

HYPOTHERMIA—A drop in body temperature.

FROSTBITE—Freezing of the skin.

SHOCK—A life-threatening condition in which the body's functions slow down.

DIRECT PRESSURE—A method of controlling bleeding by placing a clean cloth over a wound and pressing on it firmly.

CAROTID PULSE—The heartbeat you can feel on either side of your neck.

CARDIAC—Dealing with the heart.

SEIZURE—A sudden attack of illness often due to epilepsy or allergic reaction.

Seek and Find

A	T	C	H	H	E	R	K	W	A	I	W	A	E	K	N	N	I	A	O	S	I	N	T	U	P	Q	D
P	B	I	F	Y	D	G	C	E	S	P	L	S	C	T	C	I	D	U	T	T	R	E	L	P	S	I	R
I	E	R	S	P	E	F	U	D	D	E	L	H	P	I	I	O	A	J	A	C	K	H	K	P	R	C	I
E	V	N	O	O	S	T	H	A	E	T	N	O	O	L	R	B	N	G	R	S	S	U	J	E	E	H	N
N	O	E	R	T	F	S	I	R	H	T	O	C	N	R	A	S	T	O	C	A	E	G	C	E	K	L	O
B	E	H	H	H	E	E	V	E	A	S	X	K	T	E	H	E	B	S	I	K	L	T	N	O	E	W	N
E	S	A	N	E	K	N	K	S	J	K	L	M	I	N	T	S	E	D	O	N	P	G	S	Z	Z	P	R
C	A	U	E	R	U	S	E	L	W	I	T	C	H	T	O	F	P	B	G	R	L	I	G	E	N	N	I
S	E	A	R	M	D	A	C	U	K	H	I	O	E	T	E	N	E	S	E	Z	F	C	I	L	S	I	S
S	B	I	G	I	P	I	N	P	H	O	S	U	S	A	T	S	N	S	I	V	A	L	V	E	T	Y	X
I	E	R	T	A	A	U	T	D	T	F	E	D	L	C	L	Y	S	A	Y	L	K	A	A	P	T	W	T
C	I	I	A	R	R	E	N	I	O	E	N	U	A	L	V	U	R	B	S	M	A	H	E	E	C	T	T
N	O	L	Z	O	N	G	E	T	E	A	L	I	B	O	R	A	A	C	L	I	P	S	C	A	S	V	F
T	S	T	N	U	W	A	R	O	S	L	D	A	K	E	Y	N	B	Y	H	P	R	U	I	I	L	L	E
O	B	E	A	H	R	O	M	R	O	R	W	R	E	V	U	E	N	A	M	H	C	I	L	M	I	E	H
A	R	L	D	E	A	E	X	A	A	R	O	N	K	C	I	A	S	H	I	L	A	M	U	Q	V	S	K
R	P	J	U	N	T	E	U	C	Y	K	A	D	A	A	R	H	D	N	E	E	M	P	W	A	H	W	E
S	C	E	I	O	V	G	O	O	P	P	N	O	E	J	E	O	N	A	W	H	A	S	E	K	W	N	N
S	U	S	D	E	R	Y	D	B	D	L	A	Y	M	S	I	D	S	L	E	I	H	R	R	T	O	S	C

A MATTER OF LIFE AND DEATH (CH-76)

STROKES

A stroke occurs when the flow of blood to the brain is blocked, causing brain cells to die. One of the most common causes of a stroke is a blood clot that blocks an artery.

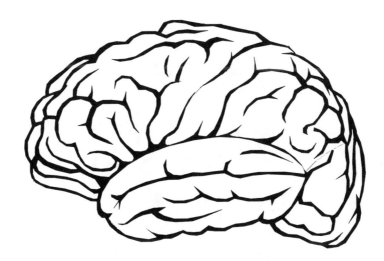

STROKE WARNING SIGNS

1. Sudden, temporary weakness or numbness of the face, arm, and/or leg on one side of the body.
2. Slurred speech, or inability to speak or understand.
3. Blurred vision or loss of vision, mainly in one eye.
4. Dizziness, unsteadiness, or sudden falls.

A MATTER OF LIFE AND DEATH (CH-77)

HEART ATTACKS

A heart attack is when the coronary arteries become clogged with fatty deposits (made up mostly of cholesterol) which eventually causes them to narrow. This causes the flow of blood to certain areas of the heart to decrease or stop which damages the heart muscle. Sometimes a total blockage of the artery causes part of the heart to be denied blood and oxygen. This is known as a heart attack.

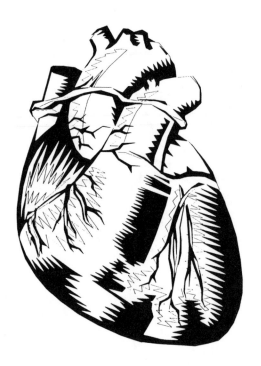

HEART ATTACK WARNING SIGNS

1. Pressure, tightening, squeezing pain in the chest lasting for more than two minutes.
2. Pain that spreads to the shoulders, neck, jaws, back, or arms.
3. Shortness of breath, dizziness, nausea, sweating, and/or fainting

A MATTER OF LIFE AND DEATH (CH-78)

CHOKING

When an airway is blocked by food or other foreign matter, unconsciousness and stoppage of breathing and heartbeat may occur. When breathing stops, death can occur since the heart, brain, and organs are deprived of vital oxygen. This is known as choking.

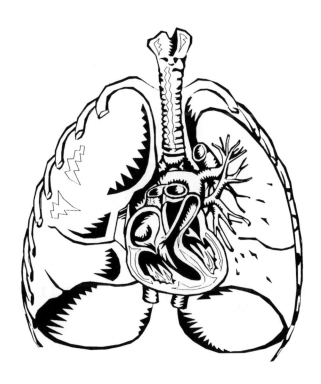

CHOKING WARNING SIGNS

1. Inability to speak or cry.
2. Grasping the neck between the thumb and fingers (the universal distress signal for choking).
3. Difficulty breathing or inability to breathe.
4. Possible bluish-color to the lips, skin, or fingernails.

Name _____   **Date** _____

EMERGENCY HANDBOOK (CH-79)

DIRECTIONS: Fill in all the information requested and cut out the pages. Staple the pages together to form your own personal emergency handbook.

EMERGENCY HANDBOOK

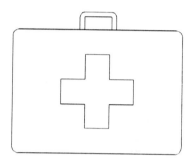

Name _____

Emergency Phone Numbers:
Ambulance _____
Police _____
Fire _____
Doctor _____
Father's Work _____
Mother's Work _____
Poison _____
Neighbor _____

1. Say: THIS IS AN EMERGENCY.
2. Calmly state the problem.
3. Explain the condition of the victim.
4. Tell what is being done.
5. Give your address and directions.
6. Give your phone number.
7. *STAY ON THE LINE UNTIL THE OTHER PARTY HANGS UP!*

GENERAL INSTRUCTIONS

1. Check the situation for immediate dangers. Do not put your safety at risk.
2. Tap the victim on the shoulder and shout, "Are you OK?" If the victim does not respond, shout for help.
3. If the person is unconscious, check to see if he or she is breathing and has a pulse.
4. If there is no breathing, no pulse, or severe bleeding, treat these conditions first.
5. Call or send someone to call for medical help.
6. Stay with the victim until help arrives.
7. Treat for shock.

VICTIM ISN'T BREATHING

Signs: No breathing movements; bluish lips, tongue, and fingernails; enlarged pupils.
Action: Perform RESCUE BREATHING
(explain below)

_____
_____
_____
_____
_____
_____
_____
_____
_____

Name _____ Date _____

EMERGENCY HANDBOOK (2) (CH-80)

VICTIM IS CHOKING

Signs: Victim cannot speak or cough.
Action: Perform the HEIMLICH MANEUVER
(explain below)

_____
_____
_____
_____
_____
_____
_____
_____
_____

NOTE: If the victim can speak or cough, do not interfere with the person's attempts to cough up the object.

VICTIM IS BLEEDING SEVERELY

Action: Apply DIRECT PRESSURE
(explain below)

_____
_____
_____
_____
_____
_____
_____
_____
_____

NOTE: To avoid the transmission of any infectious diseases, do not come in direct contact with the victim's blood.

TREATMENT FOR SHOCK

Signs: Pale, moist, cold, skin; weak or absent pulse; shallow irregular breathing; and enlarged pupils.

Action:
1. Keep the victim calm and quiet.
2. Place the victim on his/her back and elevate the feet 8 to 12 inches.
3. Maintain the victim's normal body temperature.
4. DO NOT give the victim any food or drink.
5. GET MEDICAL HELP IMMEDIATELY!

NOTES

ANSWER KEYS
TO
REPRODUCIBLES

NAME THE PRODUCT (CH-2)

DIRECTIONS: Listed below are some advertising slogans, or descriptions. Can you name the products described? Place your answer in the blank.

DIET PEPSI 1. The soft drink that states, "You got the right one, baby...uh, huh!"

ENERGIZER BATTERIES 2. A bunny appears on the TV screen as the announcer says, "It keeps going and going and going..."

CHUNKY 3. "Soup so big, it eats like a meal."

EGGOS 4. A family fights over waffles shouting, "Leggo my _____ !"

NIKE 5. "JUST DO IT!"

JELL-O 6. "There's always room for _____ ?" this gelatin dessert.

BURGER KING 7. A fast food restaurant that says you can have it "your way, right away!"

GREY POUPON 8. A man needing mustard for his sandwich rolls down the window to his Rolls Royce and asks, "Pardon me, but would you have any _____ ?"

FORD 9. A car company that asks, "Have you driven a _____ , lately?"

TOYOTA 10. A car company where its buyers jump into the air and exclaim, "I love what you do for me, _____ "

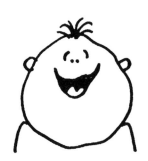

"Ummm .....
is the answer
Wendy's ?"

AD TECHNIQUES (CH-10)

DIRECTIONS: Listed below are some commonly used advertising methods. Match the ad described with the technique by placing the correct letter in the blank.

TECHNIQUES:

NOSTALGIA: Plainfolks, back-to nature, just the way grandma used to make it, back in the good old days.

BANDWAGON: Everyone who is anyone is buying this product. Don't be the only one without it. Don't be left out!

TRANSFER/FANTASY: Superheros, white knights, green giants, super athletes, beautiful people, rich people are featured. Advertisers hope that the consumer will tend to transfer these qualities to the products and themselves and purchase the item.

HUMOR: People may tend to remember an ad if it makes them laugh and may purchase the product because of the positive association with it.

SENSE APPEAL: Sounds or pictures that appeal to the senses are featured.

STATISTICS: People tend to be impressed with "facts" and statistics even if they have little or no meaning.

TESTIMONIAL: Important or well-known people testify that they use the product and so should you.

MATCHING:

__F__ 1. "Lose weight the way 6 million Americans have. It's the method 3 out of 4 doctors recommend."

__B__ 2. A cool, sparkling soft drink sits next to a hot, sizzling cheeseburger.

__D__ 3. A famous actor says that he buys a product and recommends it to everyone.

__E__ 4. Lemonade is served on the back porch of a house situated near an old fishin' pond.

__G__ 5. "Buy your next car at Crazy Joe's, where everyone gets the best deal around!"

__A__ 6. A person falls down a flight of steps and says, "It's the kind of soft drink you could fall for!"

__C__ 7. A woman driving in her new convertible runs her hands through her beautiful blonde hair to show how great Shimmer Shampoo works.

A. Humor
B. Sense Appeal
C. Transfer/Fantasy
D. Testimonial
E. Nostalgia
F. Statistics
G. Bandwagon

THE SKIN YOU'RE IN (CH-13)

DIRECTIONS: Take the skin quiz below to discover how much you know about your skin. Write an *X* in the correct box.

	TRUE	FALSE
1. The largest organ in the body is the skin.	☒	☐
2. The most effective over-the-counter (OTC) treatment for acne is to use products that contain benzoyl peroxide.	☒	☐
3. Medicated soaps are a great treatment for acne because the medication seeps into the pores.	☐	☒
4. Acne occurs when the skin pores become clogged with dead skin cells and dirt.	☒	☐
5. Products containing lanolin are best to use if you have acne.	☐	☒
6. Acne is caused by eating fatty foods and chocolate.	☐	☒
7. Antibacterial soaps are excellent in the treatment of acne.	☐	☒
8. If you have acne, it is best to use water-based cosmetics or no cosmetics at all.	☒	☐
9. The most active sebaceous (oil-producing) glands are located in the scalp.	☒	☐
10. Look for products containing sulfur, resorcinol, or salicylic acid to treat the more severe cases of acne.	☐	☒

DO YOU CARE ABOUT YOUR HAIR? (CH-15)

DIRECTIONS: How much do you know about hair care? Place a *T* for TRUE or an *F* for FALSE in the blank?

F   1. Only shampoos that produce a great deal of suds or lather clean well.

T   2. Using mild dishwashing liquid to shampoo your hair will not damage your hair.

T   3. Ingredients such as egg, lemon juice, and herbs are of no special benefit to the hair.

F   4. Certain types of shampoo will mend split ends.

T   5. Surfactants are chemicals in shampoo that can grab hold of dirt and oil and then attract water to wash them away.

F   6. Shampoos for oily hair contain less detergent than those for dry hair.

T   7. Washing your hair several times per week, no matter which shampoo you use, generally keeps dandruff under control.

T   8. If you do experience "flaking" of the scalp, a shampoo containing selenium may help.

F   9. For shampoos to be safe, they should be "pH balanced."

F   10. To have clean, "healthy" hair, you need to purchase a well-known hair care system.

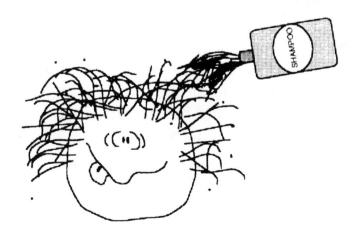

I'VE GOT A SECRET! (CH-20)

DIRECTIONS: Shown below is a "quack" advertisement for a fictitious product. Circle all the things in this ad that would make it quackery. Refer to the SIGNS OF QUACKERY (CH-19) list if you need help.

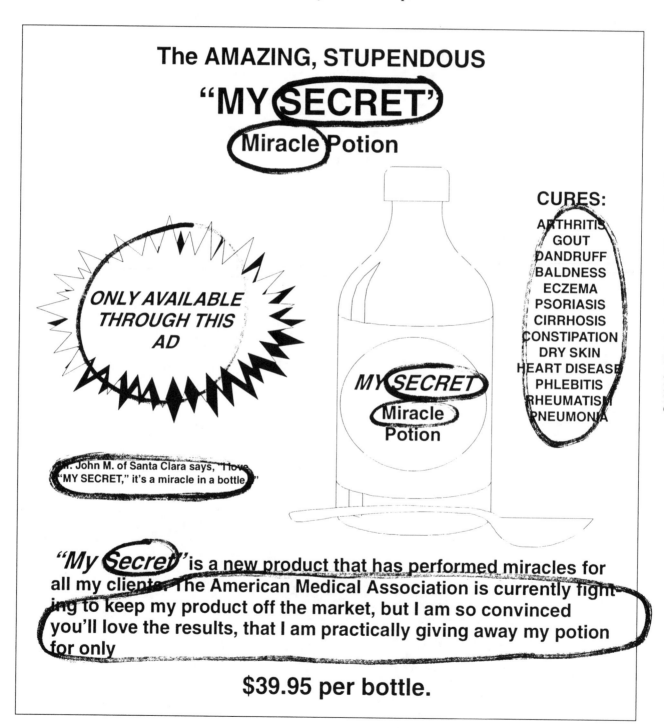

MEDICAL QUACKERY (CH-23)

DIRECTIONS: Unscramble the words to form a list of terms dealing with common forms of medical quackery.

1. ACCENR   **CANCER**   abnormal growth of cells

2. LPCEAOB   **PLACEBO**   substance that has no medical value

3. SITIRHTRA   **ARTHRITIS**   condition that causes aching and pain in the joints

4. GGANI   **AGING**   growing old

5. EIWHGT   **WEIGHT**   heaviness

6. DIAS   **AIDS**   acquired immune deficiency syndrome

7. LDABSSNE   **BALDNESS**   hair loss

8. LESRWKNI   **WRINKLES**   caused by aging or ultraviolet rays

9. DOOF DAFS   **FOOD FADS**   schemes that feature food, diets, or diet supplements

10. STUB VDEELPORES   breast enhancers
       BUST DEVELOPERS

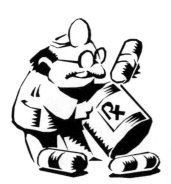

"I bet this stuff will grow hair..."

NOW WHAT DO I DO? (CH-27)

DIRECTIONS: For each scenario listed below, match it with the agency or group that is most likely able to help. Place the letter of the BEST choice in the blank. Refer to the worksheet "NADER'S RAIDERS" (CH 25-26) for help in determining what each agency does.

a. BBB (Better Business Bureau)
b. Small-Claims Court
c. CIC (Consumer Information Center)
d. CPSC (Consumer Product Safety Commission)
e. FDA (Food and Drug Administration)
f. FTC (Federal Trade Commission)
g. FSQS (Food and Safety Quality Service)

__d__ 1. The head fell off of the doll you bought for your sister, exposing a sharp, jagged piece of metal.

__a__ 2. A local business placed an ad in a local paper, and you believe it is false advertising.

__a__ 3. You want to check out the complaint record of a local business.

__c__ 4. You would like a catalogue of consumer information.

__e__ 5. You have a severe skin rash and blistering after using a new brand of deodorant.

__b__ 6. After taking your new car to a car wash, you notice about $500 worth of damage to the paint and trim. The owner refuses to pay for repairs, but you are certain that it is the fault of the car wash.

__d__ 7. The electric razor that you bought gives you an electric shock each time you attempt to use it.

__e__ 8. You purchase a can of fruit that is contaminated by worms.

__e__ 9. A new type of eye mascara causes a burning sensation in your eyes.

__g__ 10. You purchase chicken that does not look or taste like chicken. You believe that the package is labeled incorrectly.

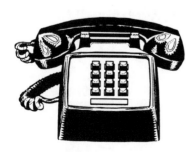

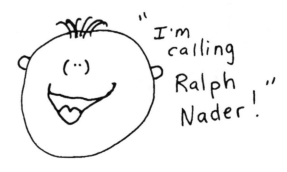

"I'm calling Ralph Nader!"

CONSUMER CROSSWORD (CH-33)

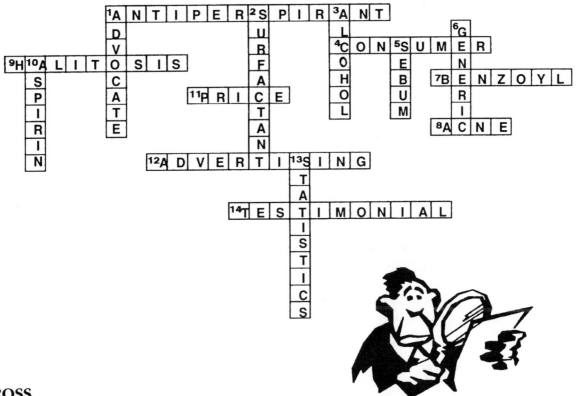

ACROSS

1. A product that helps control underarm perspiration
4. A person who buys or uses goods or services
7. An effective OTC ingredient to fight acne is _____ peroxide
8. A skin disorder
9. Bad breath
11. Cost or _____
12. All the methods a manufacturer uses to get your attention for its product
14. A method of advertising where a famous or important person tells how great the product is and that you, too, should use it

DOWN

1. A person who speaks out for a position
2. A compound in shampoo that attracts oil and water and cleans your hair
3. An ingredient to avoid in mouthwash since too much can dry out the mouth
5. The oil secreted from the glands of the skin and scalp
6. Not a "brand name" drug
10. Acetylsalicylic acid
13. A method of advertising that sometimes uses insignificant facts and figures to tout the product

TEST YOUR KNOWLEDGE (CH-34)

DIRECTIONS: How knowledgeable are you about consumer health? Take the test below to find out. Place a *T* for TRUE or an *F* for FALSE in the blank to the left.

F   1. Certain types of gum can freshen your breath and whiten your teeth.

F   2. It is unsafe to use a generic brand of aspirin because it might not contain the correct ingredients.

F   3. If statistics, such as "three out of four doctors recommend this product," are used in a commercial, then the product would definitely be good.

F   4. The best way for a woman to keep herself clean is to use feminine deodorant sprays and douche regularly.

T   5. Using mouthwashes containing alcohol can actually dry out the mouth and possibly contribute to infection.

F   6. The best acne medications to use contain alcohol which helps to dry out the skin and promote healing.

T   7. Medicated soaps are a waste of money because the medication washes off when you rinse.

F   8. If a product label does not specifically say it has SUGAR in it, then it does not contain sugar.

F   9. A good diet for SAFE weight loss is to eat a lot of protein and completely cut out carbohydrates and fats.

T   10. If the ingredients on a can of beef stew are listed as follows: potatoes, peas, carrots, water, spices, and beef, then there is very little beef in the beef stew.

©1993 by The Center for Applied Research in Education

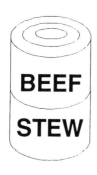

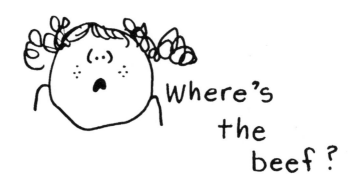

FIRE HOUSE (CH-36)

DIRECTIONS: Listed below are the three components required to have a fire. In the box are examples of fuel, heat sources, and air. Place each word in the box under the correct category. If any one component of a fire is removed, there can be no fire.

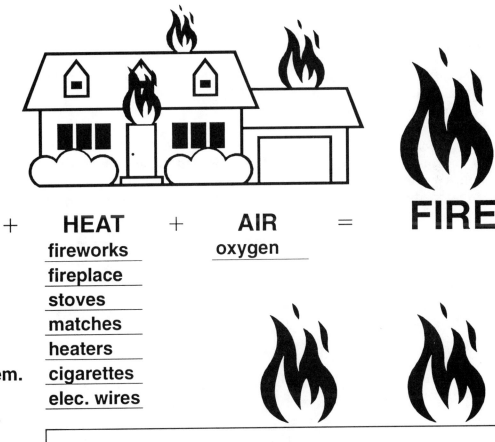

FUEL   +

coal

rags

oil

kerosene

gasoline

nail polish rem.

lighter fluid

paint thinner

paper

rub. alcohol

furn. polish

HEAT   +

fireworks

fireplace

stoves

matches

heaters

cigarettes

elec. wires

AIR   =

oxygen

FIRE

OXYGEN	GASOLINE
COAL	HEATERS
FIREWORKS	NAIL POLISH REMOVER
FIREPLACE	LIGHTER FLUID
STOVES	CIGARETTES
RAGS	ELECTRICAL WIRES
OIL	PAINT THINNER
KEROSENE	PAPER
MATCHES	RUBBING ALCOHOL
	FURNITURE POLISH

PICK YOUR POISON (CH-39)

DIRECTIONS: Listed below are the descriptions for three types of poisoning: oral, inhalation, and contact. Research the first aid for each type of poisoning and place your answers in the boxes next to each type.

ORAL POISONING

Swallowing a harmful substance, such as bleach, medicines, or poisonous plants.
<u>Signs:</u> sudden, severe stomach pain; nausea or vomiting; burns on or around the mouth; drowsiness; chemical odor on the breath; dilated or constricted pupils; container from a harmful substance nearby.

FIRST AID

Call a poison control center immediately and follow instructions. If breathing has stopped, apply rescue breathing through the nose to avoid contact with poison on the mouth.

INHALATION POISONING

Breathing dangerous gases or fumes, such as car exhaust, glue, paints, solvents, and fuels.
<u>Signs:</u> dizziness or headache followed by unconsciousness.

FIRST AID

Protect your safety first. Hold your breath and get victim to fresh air. Get medical help immediately. Loosen clothing around the neck and waist. Keep victim's airway open by tilting head.

CONTACT POISONING

Touching a dangerous substance, such as solvents, pesticides, and plants, such as poison ivy, poison oak, and poison sumac.
<u>Signs:</u> Rash, swelling, burning, itching, blisters.

FIRST AID

Remove contaminated clothing and pour large amounts of water over the skin. Wash the area with soap and water. Call a poison control center if a chemical or solvent.

WATER SAFETY UNSCRAMBLE (CH-44)

DIRECTIONS: Unscramble the jumbled words to reveal ten water safety rules. Place the unscrambled word in the blank to the right.

1. Don't swim immediately after taegni.

   eating
   _____

2. Always swim in an area where a filedgrua is present.

   lifeguard
   _____

3. Always swim with a dduby.

   buddy
   _____

4. Don't use underwater equipment unless you have been raintde.

   trained
   _____

5. Wear a lotfaatoin device when required.

   floatation
   _____

6. Never dive in an desnspvuueri or unfamiliar area.

   unsupervised
   _____

7. Never swim or dive after using laocohl or other drugs.

   alcohol
   _____

8. Do not walk on cie that may be unsafe.

   ice
   _____

9. If you are on ice that begins to crack, lie down and rwcal to shore.

   crawl
   _____

10. Learn poofdrrwongin techniques.

    drownproofing
    _____

IT WAS AN ACCIDENT! (CH-46)

DIRECTIONS: Look at the chart below that deals with the leading causes of accidental death, then answer the questions.

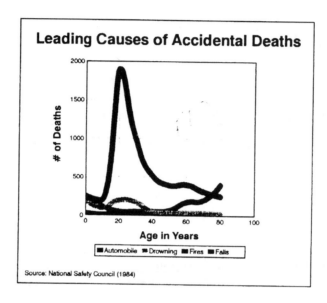

Leading Causes of Accidental Deaths

# of Deaths

Age in Years

■ Automobile ■ Drowning ■ Fires ■ Falls

Source: National Safety Council (1984)

1. According to the chart, which age group suffered the most deaths from auto accidents?

20 year olds

2. Why do you think this is the case? **Take more unnecessary risks. Have less driving experience.**

3. Which age group is most susceptible to death from falls? **Elderly**

4. Why do you think this is the case? **Less mobile, vision is worse with age.**

5. Which two age groups seem to have the most deaths from drowning?

Young children and 20 year olds.

6. Give some reasons for this. **Children unsupervised or don't know how to swim. Teenagers and young adults may use alcohol and other drugs.**

THERE'S NO PLACE LIKE HOME (CH-47)

DIRECTIONS: Look at the chart below that deals with the leading causes of accidental deaths in the home, then answer the questions.

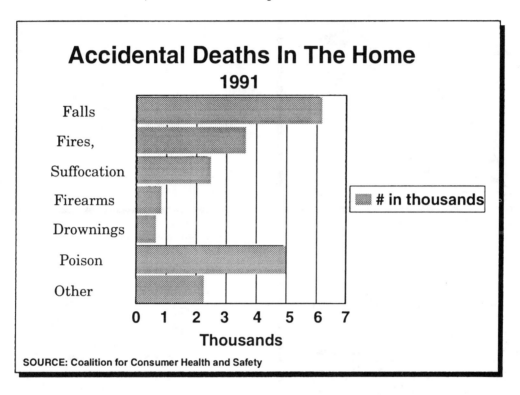

1. According to the chart, what is the leading cause of accidental death in the home?
Falls

2. What could be done to eliminate this hazard? **Keep walkways clear, don't climb on unsteady objects.**

3. What is the second leading cause of accidental home deaths? **Poison**

4. What age group do you think is most affected by this? **Young children.**

   Why? **They put unknown things into their mouths.**

5. Give examples of what you think the "other" category might include:

Heart attacks, strokes, allergic reactions, abuse, bleeding severely, electric shock.

WHAT'S WRONG WITH THIS PICTURE? (CH-58)

DIRECTIONS: On the back of this sheet, list everything wrong with each picture.

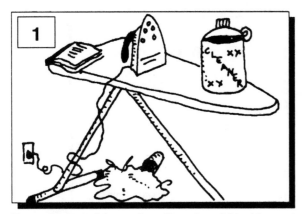

Flammable materials near iron. Frayed cord. Liquid spilled near cord.

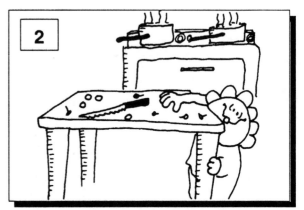

Pot handles in dangerous position. Stove unsupervised. Dangerous objects within child's reach.

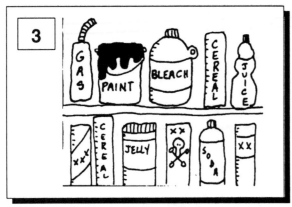

Poisonous substances stored near foods.

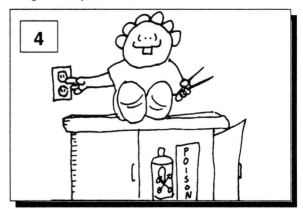

No outlet safety covers; poisons within child's reach, sharp object within child's reach. Child unsupervised.

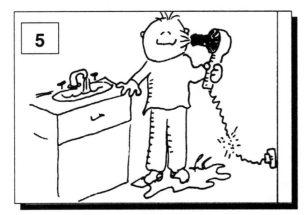

Frayed cord. Appliance used near water.

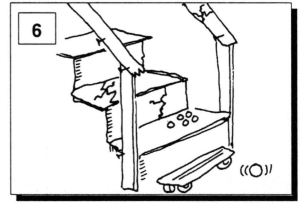

Cracked steps and railings. Dangerous objects on steps. Protruding nails.

BITES AND STINGS (CH-68)

DIRECTIONS: Match the insect or animal to the type of treatment, by placing the letter in the box surrounding each picture. Letters may be used more than once.

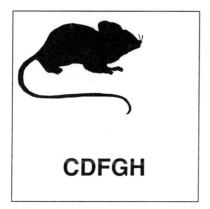

CDFGH

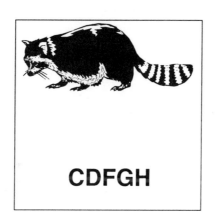

CDFGH

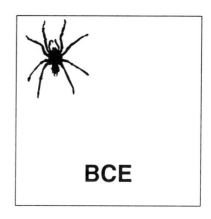

BCE

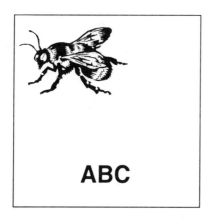

ABC

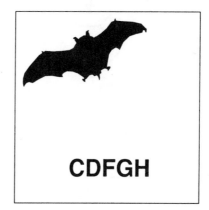

CDFGH

A. Scrape off the stinger with your fingernail, a flat piece of cardboard, or a credit card.

B. Apply ice or a paste of baking soda and water.

C. Keep the victim calm.

D. Wash with soap and water.

E. Seek immediate medical attention and treat for shock.

F. If possible, catch the animal so it can be examined for rabies. Don't risk your health to do so, however.

G. Seek medical attention and notify the health department.

H. Cover the wound with a clean, dry dressing.

BEE SAFE (CH-69)

DIRECTIONS: In the beehive, find and circle the words that explain the symptoms and signs of an allergic reaction to bee stings. Use the clues below to figure out the words.

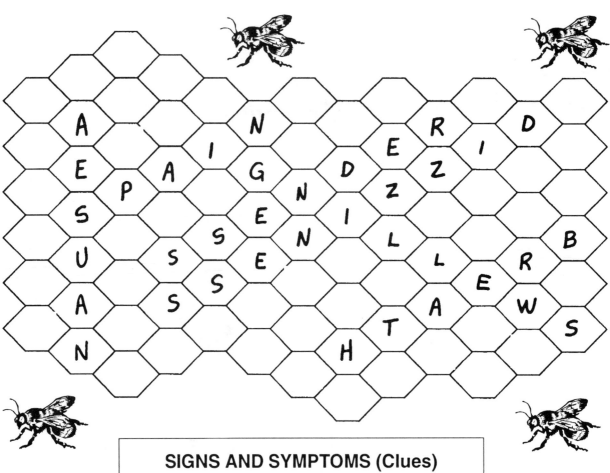

SIGNS AND SYMPTOMS (Clues)

P A I N

SHORTNESS OF B RE A T H

R E DNE S S

S W E L L I N G

D I ZZI N E S S

N A U S E A

BE A LIFESAVER! (CH-71)

DIRECTIONS: Using the words in the box, fill in the steps you should take to help someone who may be experiencing a life or death situation.

DRIVE	**PULSE**
EMERGENCY	**QUIETLY**
LICENSED	**BREATHING**
911	**TRAINED**
CPR	**SPEAK**
INTERFERE	**HEIMLICH**

1. If you are with someone who is having a heart attack or stroke, have him or her rest **quietly**.

2. Call the **emergency** medical system (EMS). This could be the fire department, an ambulance service, **911**, or other emergency number.

3. If driving the victim to the hospital would be faster, then a **licensed** driver should take the victim there. Do not let the victim **drive**.

4. If the person has no **pulse** or is not **breathing**, perform **CPR** if you are **trained**.

5. If the person is choking and can **speak**, breathe, or cough do not **interfere** unless his or her condition gets worse.

6. If the victim is choking and cannot breathe or speak, perform the **Heimlich** Maneuver if you are trained to do so.

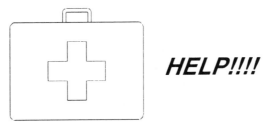

HELP!!!!

TEST YOUR FIRST AID I.Q. (CH-74)

DIRECTIONS: Place the letter of the best answer in the blank to the left.

__b__ 1. After you have rescued a person, the FIRST thing you should do is
    a. get help.
    b. check the victim's breathing.
    c. control severe bleeding.

__c__ 2. Which is not a preferred way to control bleeding?
    a. Apply direct pressure to the wound.
    b. Use pressure points.
    c. Apply a tourniquet.

__b__ 3. Which is NOT a sign of shock?
    a. Shallow, uneven breathing.
    b. The skin is dry, warm, and reddish.
    c. The pulse is weak or cannot be felt.

__c__ 4. Which is NOT a method of helping a poisoning victim?
    a. Call a poison control center or a doctor and follow instructions.
    b. Save the container of the poisonous substance and show it to the medical team when they arrive.
    c. Immediately induce vomiting.

__a__ 5. Which SHOULD be done in case of a third-degree burn?
    a. Cover the burned area with a clean dressing.
    b. Remove burned clothing.
    c. Apply ice to the burn.

__b__ 6. If you are stung by a wasp or bee, you should
    a. pull out the stinger with a pair of tweezers.
    b. scrape across the stinger with a piece of cardboard or credit card.
    c. leave the stinger alone and apply ice.

__c__ 7. If a person suffers a sprained ankle, you should
    a. raise the sprained part and apply heat.
    b. lower the sprained part and apply ice.
    c. raise the sprained part and apply cold packs.

__a__ 8. First aid for a nosebleed is
    a. sit, lean forward, and pinch the nose firmly for 5 minutes.
    b. lie down and pinch the nose shut for 5 minutes.
    c. tilt the head back and apply ice to the back of the neck.

__b__ 9. If a person faints, you should
    a. pour water over his or her face.
    b. raise his or her legs 8 to 12 inches.
    c. try to help him or her to a standing position.

__b__ 10. The Good Samaritan Law says that anyone who tries to help in an emergency
    a. must be certified in first aid.
    b. cannot be sued unless he or she knowingly acted unsafely.

©1993 by The Center for Applied Research in Education

EMERGENCY TERMS YOU SHOULD KNOW (CH-75)

DIRECTIONS: Review the words below, then find them in the Seek and Find. Words may be vertical, horizontal, or diagonal, frontwards and backwards.

CPR (Cardiopulmonary Resuscitation)—A technique in which breathing is restored by mouth-to-mouth resuscitation and heartbeat is restored by chest compression.

HEIMLICH MANEUVER—A method of helping a choking victim by performing under-the-diaphragm abdominal thrusts to expel an object blocking the trachea (windpipe).

HYPOTHERMIA—A drop in body temperature.

FROSTBITE—Freezing of the skin.

SHOCK—A life-threatening condition in which the body's functions slow down.

DIRECT PRESSURE—A method of controlling bleeding by placing a clean cloth over a wound and pressing on it firmly.

CAROTID PULSE—The heartbeat you can feel on either side of your neck.

CARDIAC—Dealing with the heart.

SEIZURE—A sudden attack of illness often due to epilepsy or allergic reaction.

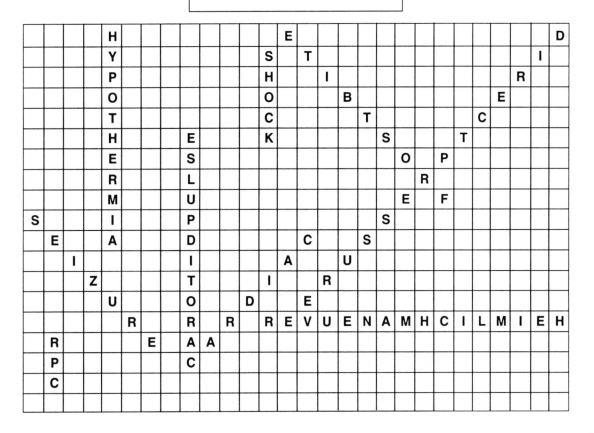

Seek and Find